Do you want to be an Athletic Trainer?

Marsha Grant-Ford, ATC,PhD and Jonathan Ford

Printed by Spyder Publications in the United States of America ISBN-13: 978-0692386767

Credits

Alison Savoia, graphic designer

Photo Credits

Jennifer Carda front cover
Alison Savoia back cover
Courtesy of Said Hamden page 2
Marsha Grant-Ford pages 3,4,7,12,14-16,18,21,23-26,27r,30l,32 top l
Sarah Kilian-Meneghin pages 6,8,9,20,30R,34,35,38,39
Courtesy of Michigan State Athletic Communications pages 10,27l
Courtesy of Miyuki Hattori page 11
Courtesy of Damien Bziukiewicz page 13
Courtesy of Pectus Services (www.pectusservices.com) page 17
Courtesy of Paceguard (www.paceguard.com) page 16
Courtesy of Rose Snyder page 22
Courtesy of Roger Hinds page 27c
Courtesy of Eric Sugarman page 28l
Courtesy of Nancy Goldsmith-Perry page 29l
Courtesy of Roberta Kuechler page 29r
Courtesy of Dawn Gulick page 32 top r
Courtesy of Chelsea Davis pages 32 bottom l & c,33l
Courtesy of Jeremy Marra page 32 bottom r
Courtesy of Erika Zimmerman page 36

**The authors also acknowledge International Sports Training Camp & Montclair State
University for their assistance in creating this book**.

Certified athletic trainers are health care professionals who work with doctors to help keep active people moving at work and at play.

3

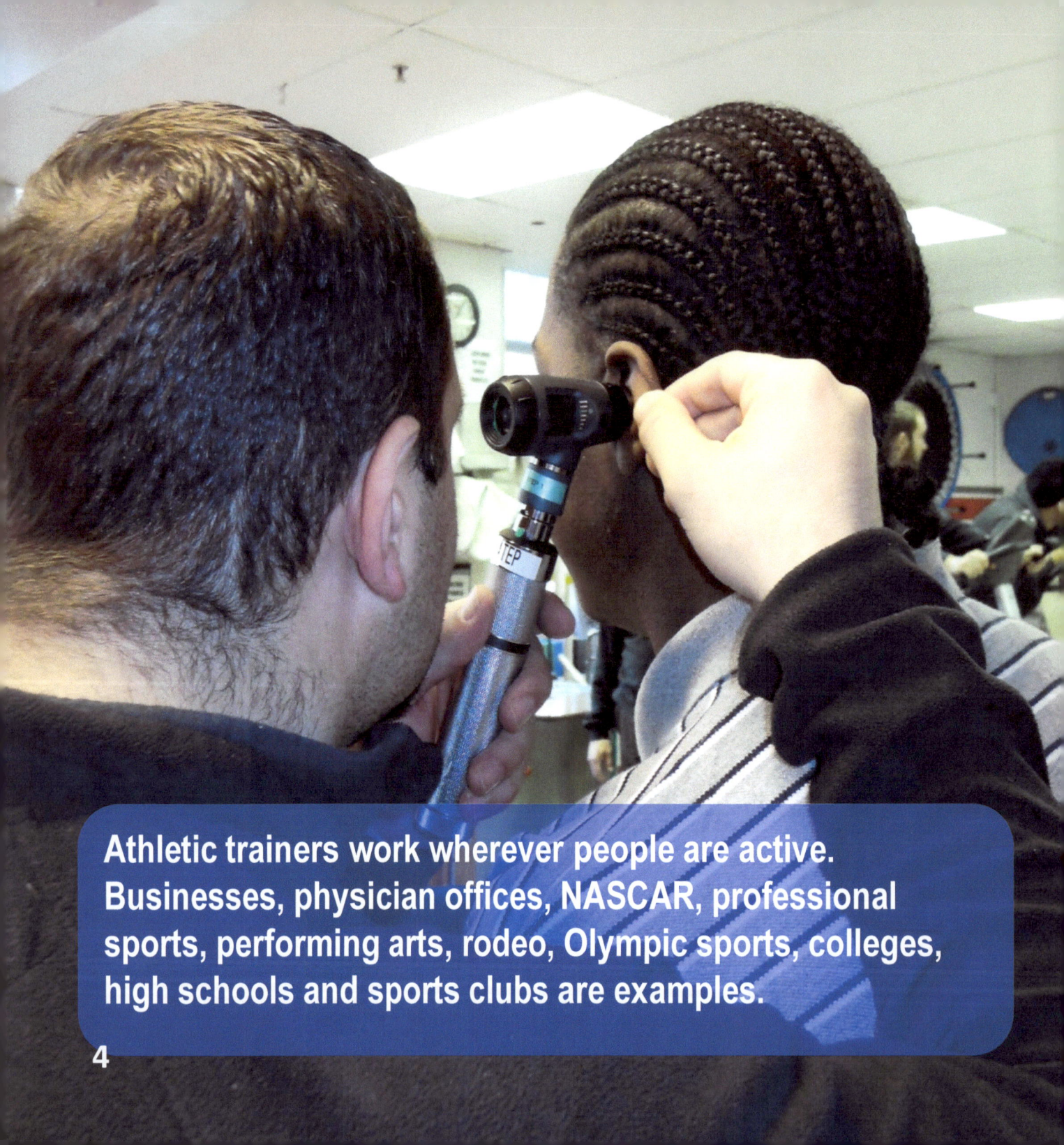

Athletic trainers work wherever people are active. Businesses, physician offices, NASCAR, professional sports, performing arts, rodeo, Olympic sports, colleges, high schools and sports clubs are examples.

Athletic trainers love what they do because they want to help people stay healthy and play healthy.

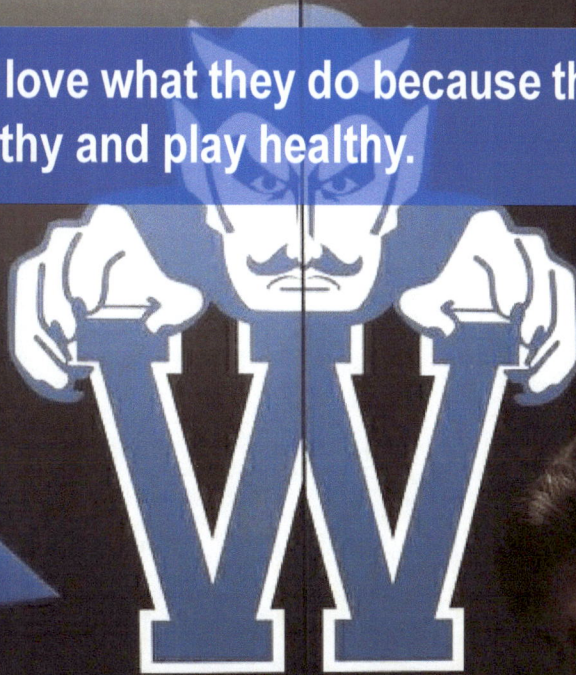

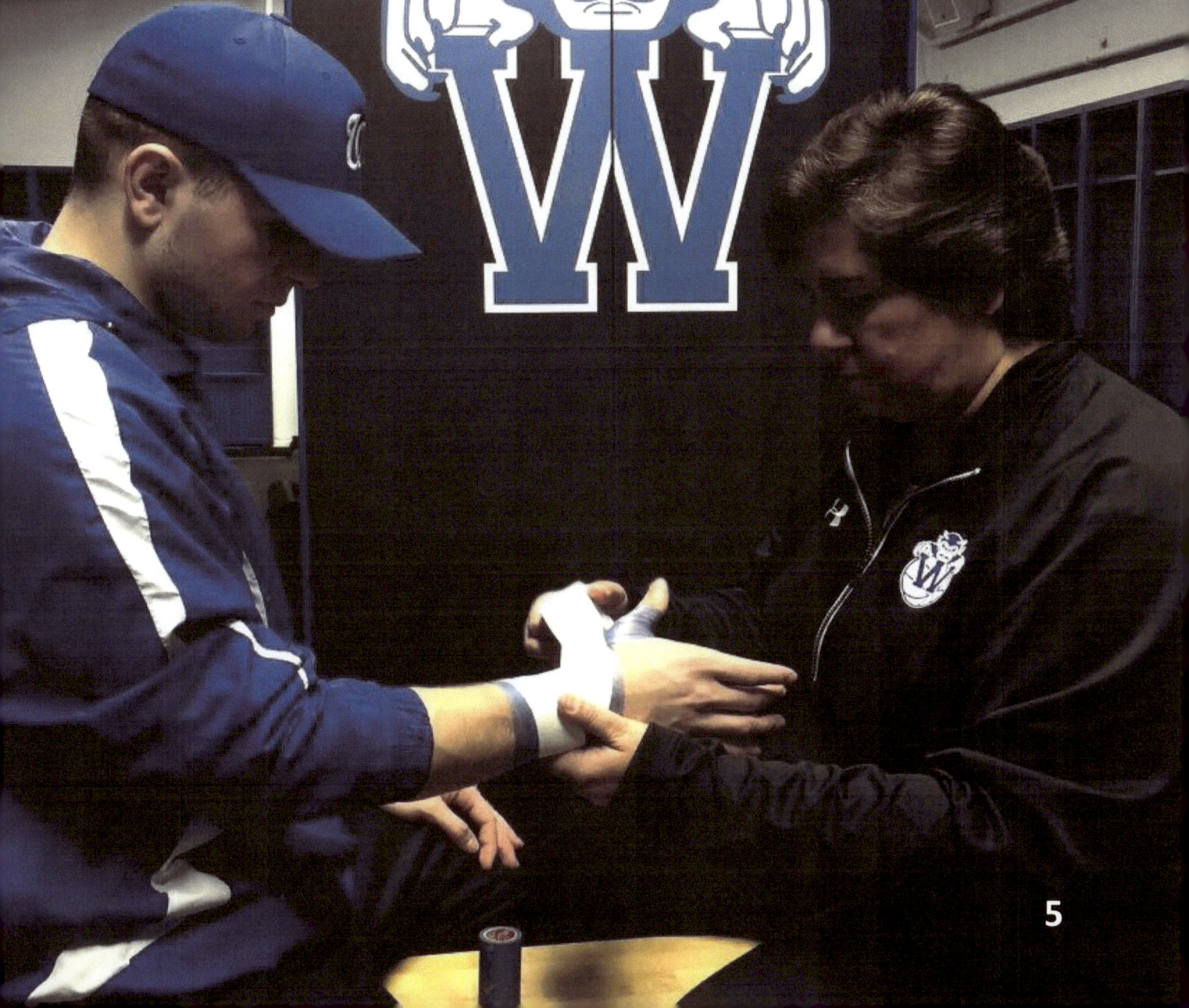

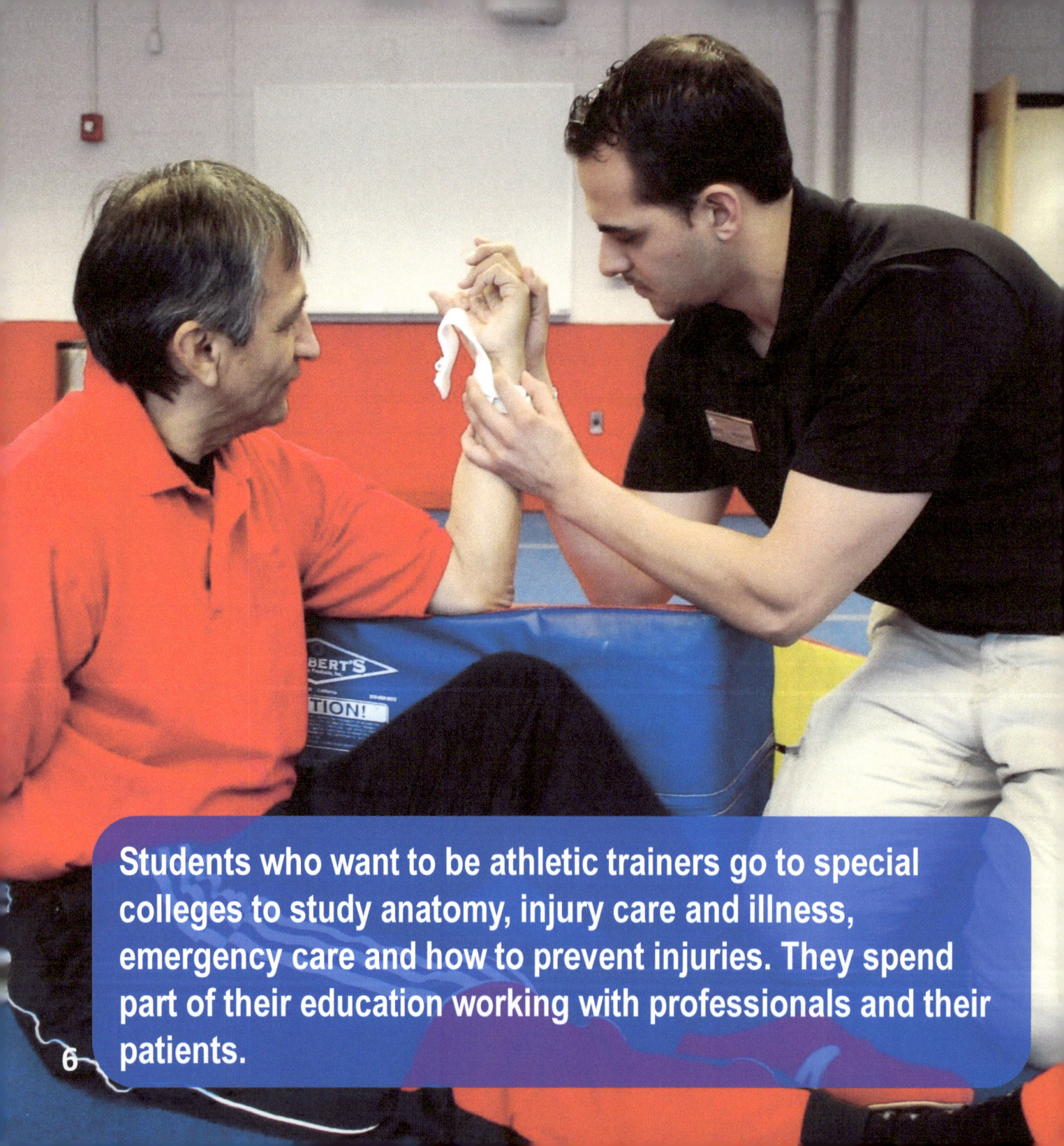

Students who want to be athletic trainers go to special colleges to study anatomy, injury care and illness, emergency care and how to prevent injuries. They spend part of their education working with professionals and their patients.

This soccer player had to use her asthma medication today during practice. The athletic trainer listens to the lungs with a stethoscope to tell how well the medication is working until it is safe for her to practice again. As you can see, she felt better later!

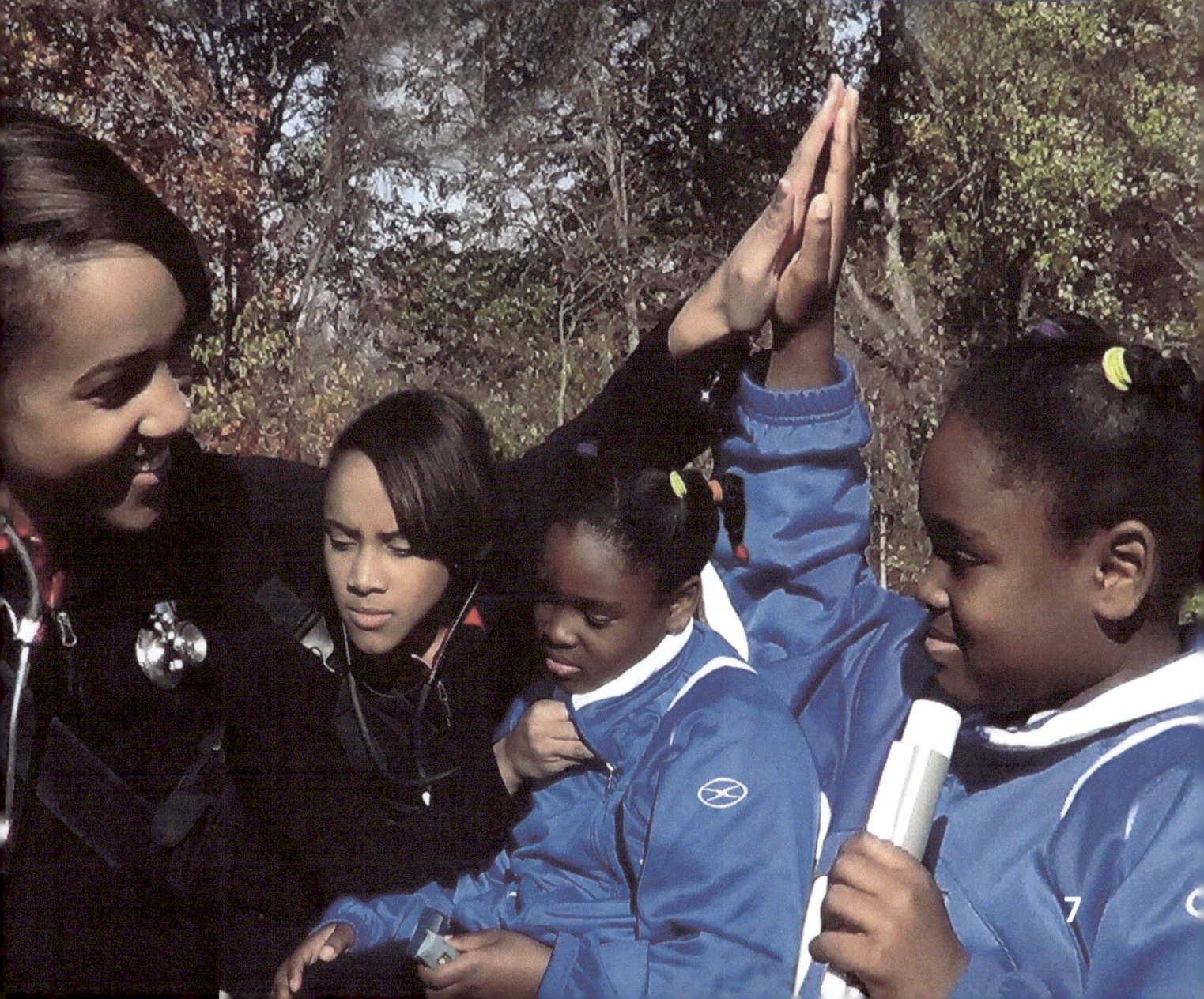

This athletic trainer is also a professor. He is teaching an athletic training student how to listen to a patient's lungs with a stethoscope.

Look, this special stethoscope has two sets of ear pieces so they both can hear the same sounds.

Athletic trainers use interpreters when they do not speak the same language as their patients. This athletic trainer is examining a Deaf athlete's painful shin injury.

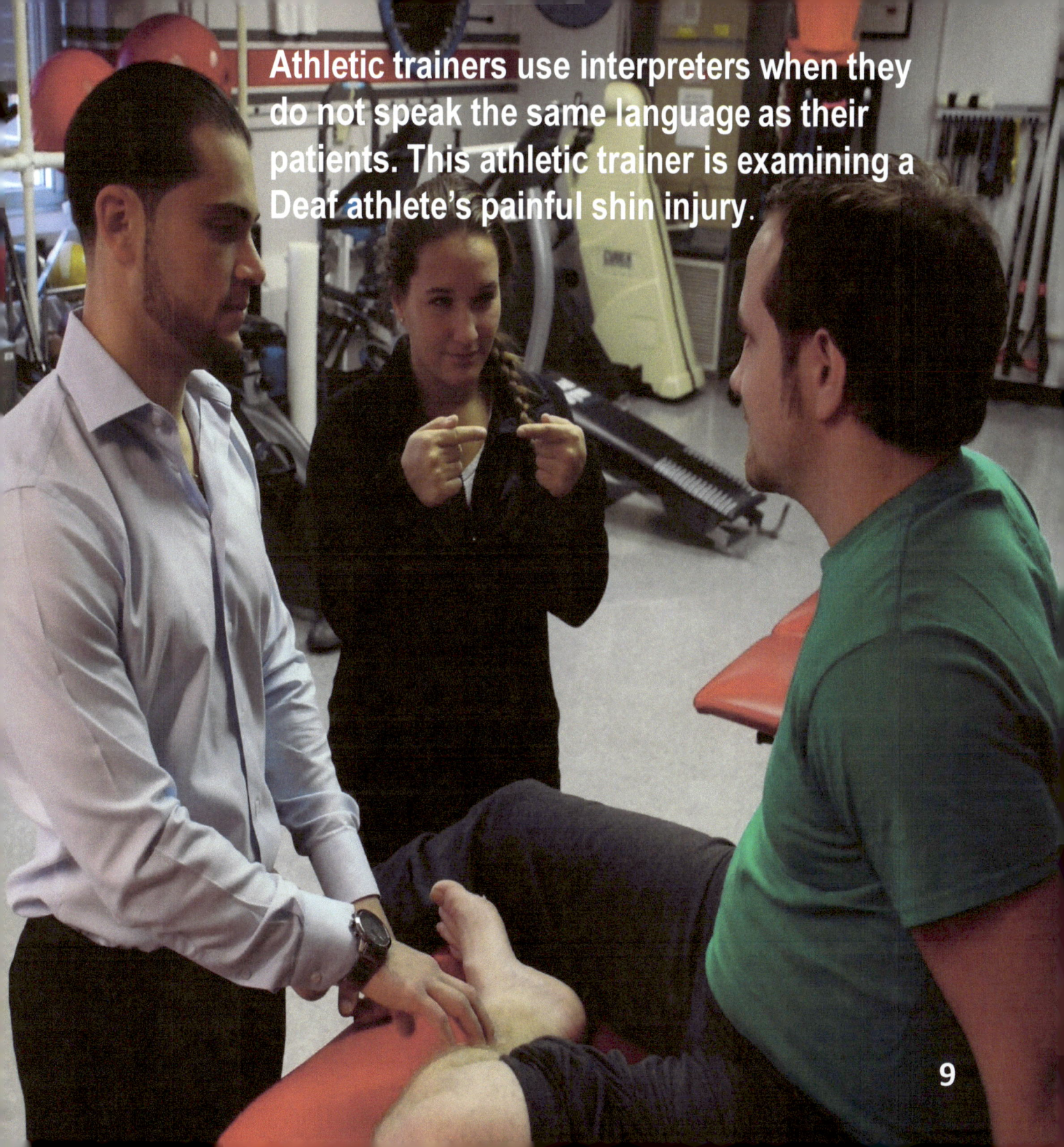

9

This athletic trainer is working to control the patient's nosebleed during a basketball game. When caring for wounds, athletic trainers wear gloves to protect the patient and themselves from germs.

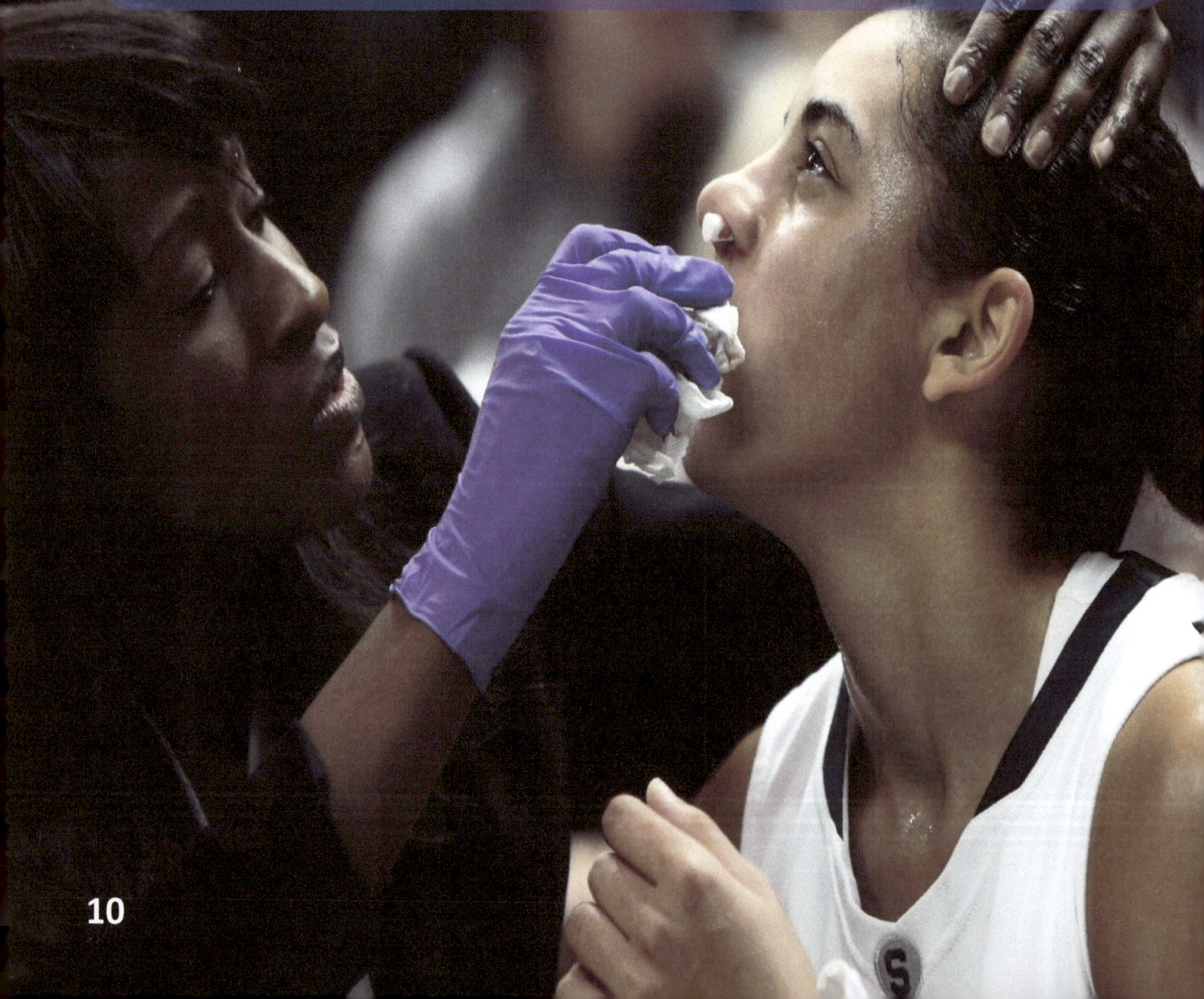

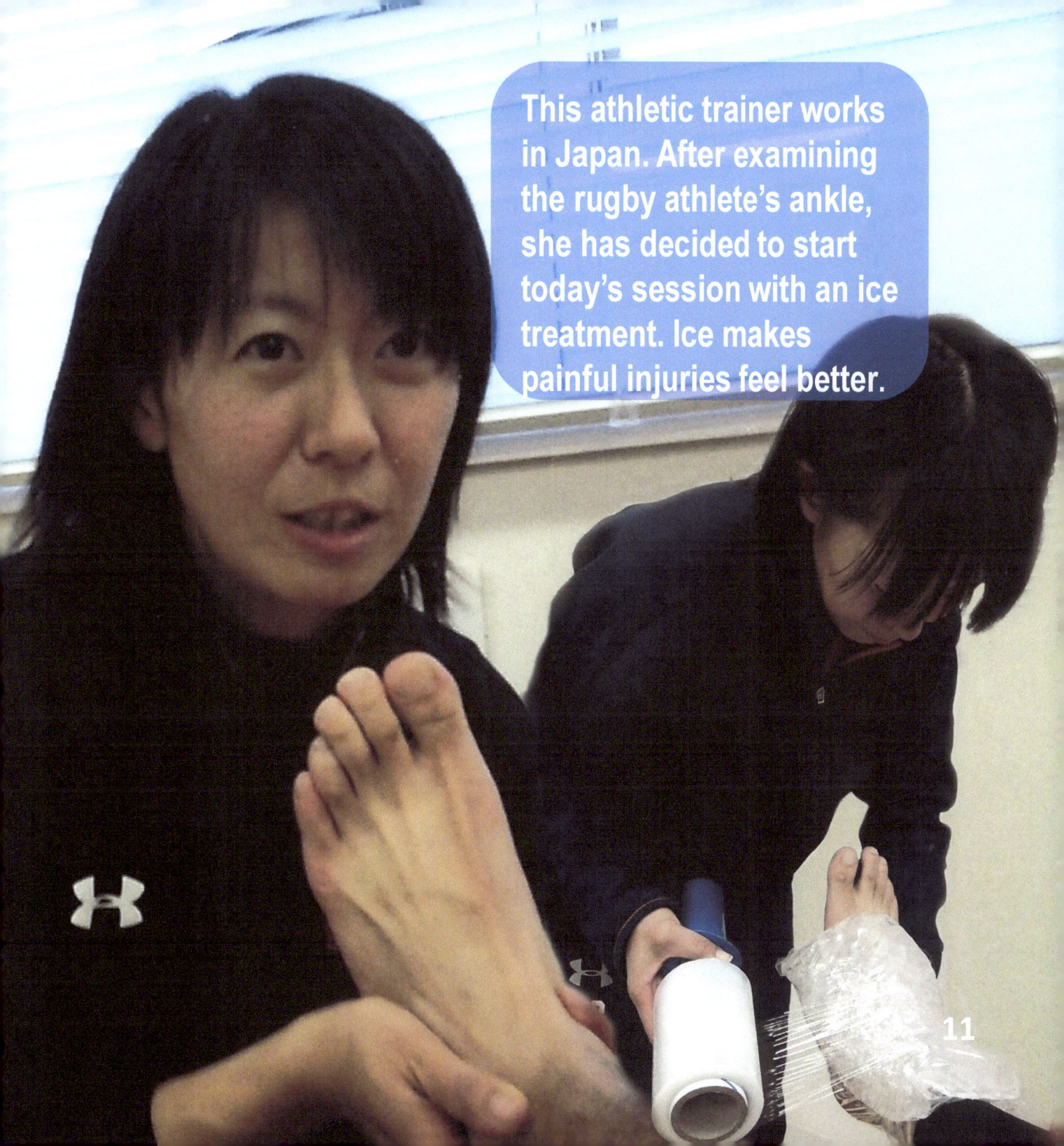

This athletic trainer works in Japan. After examining the rugby athlete's ankle, she has decided to start today's session with an ice treatment. Ice makes painful injuries feel better.

11

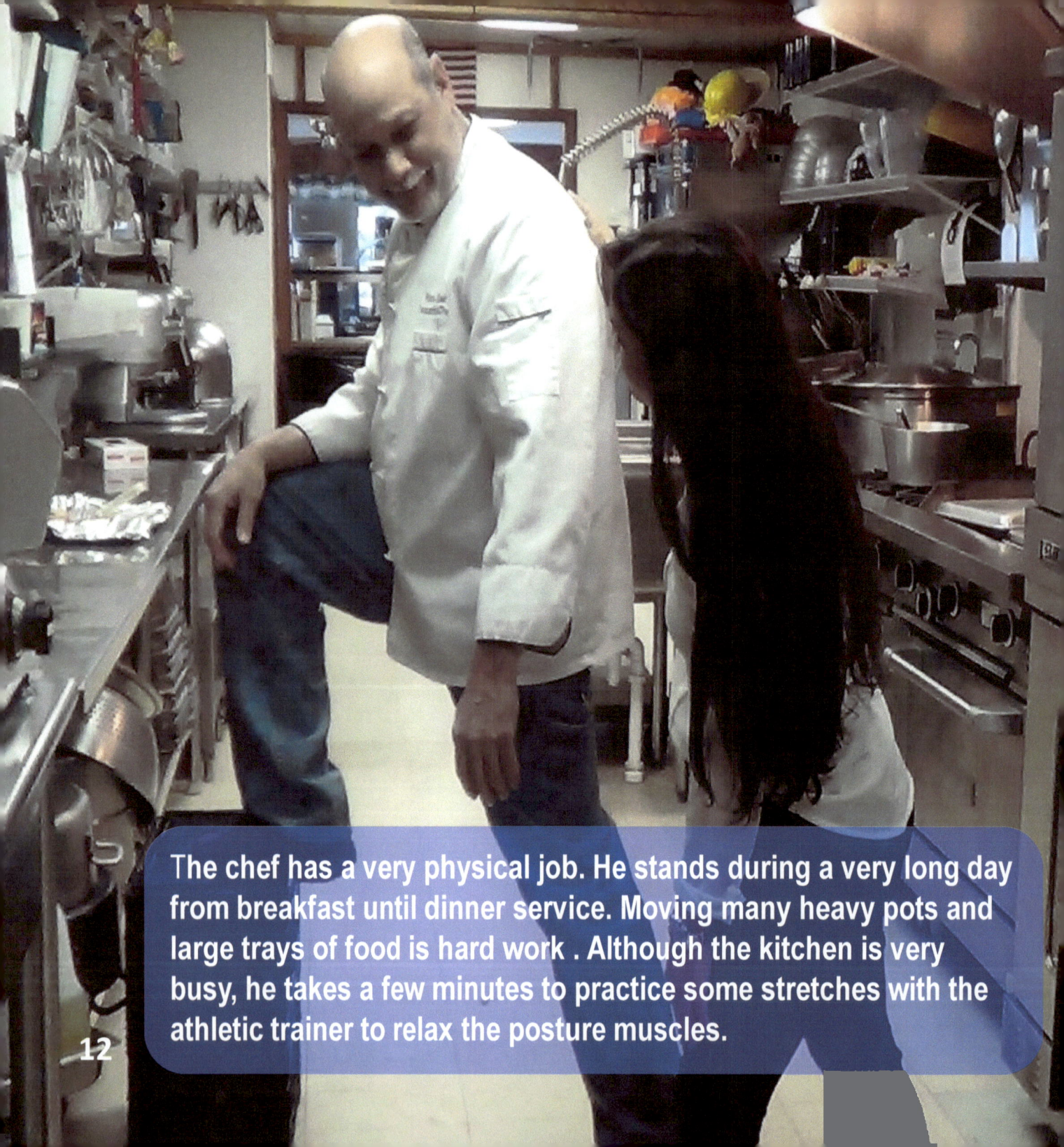

The chef has a very physical job. He stands during a very long day from breakfast until dinner service. Moving many heavy pots and large trays of food is hard work . Although the kitchen is very busy, he takes a few minutes to practice some stretches with the athletic trainer to relax the posture muscles.

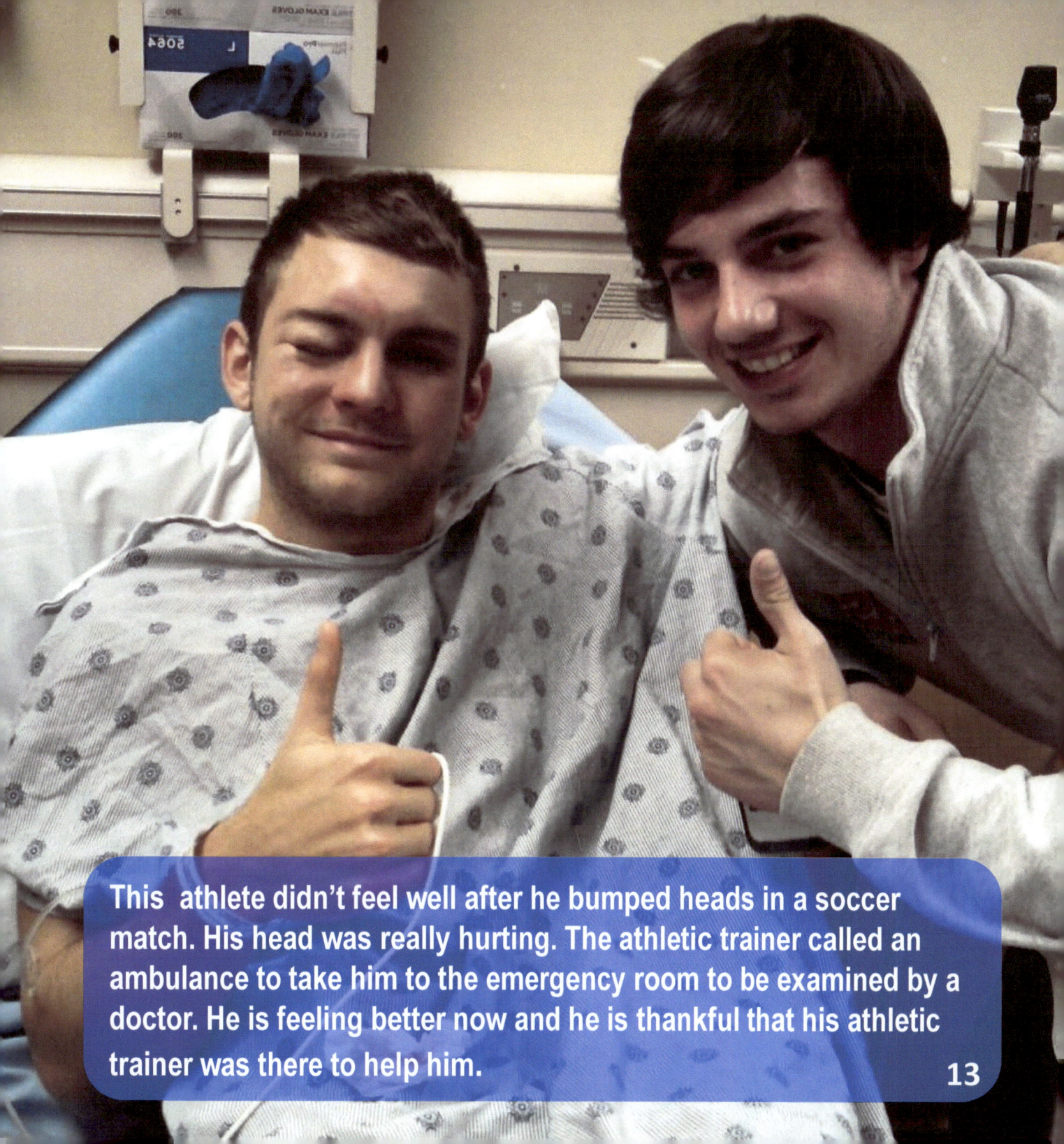

This athlete didn't feel well after he bumped heads in a soccer match. His head was really hurting. The athletic trainer called an ambulance to take him to the emergency room to be examined by a doctor. He is feeling better now and he is thankful that his athletic trainer was there to help him.

13

This patient hurt his finger playing gaga ball. The athletic trainer placed a splint on it to protect it.

The parents are learning how to care for this injury until the doctor's appointment.

This athlete had surgery last week to repair a torn knee ligament. Athletic trainers help people get better with different treatments and special exercises or stretches. The athletic trainer is helping her with an exercise to help the knee move better. This is called rehabilitation, or rehab, for short.

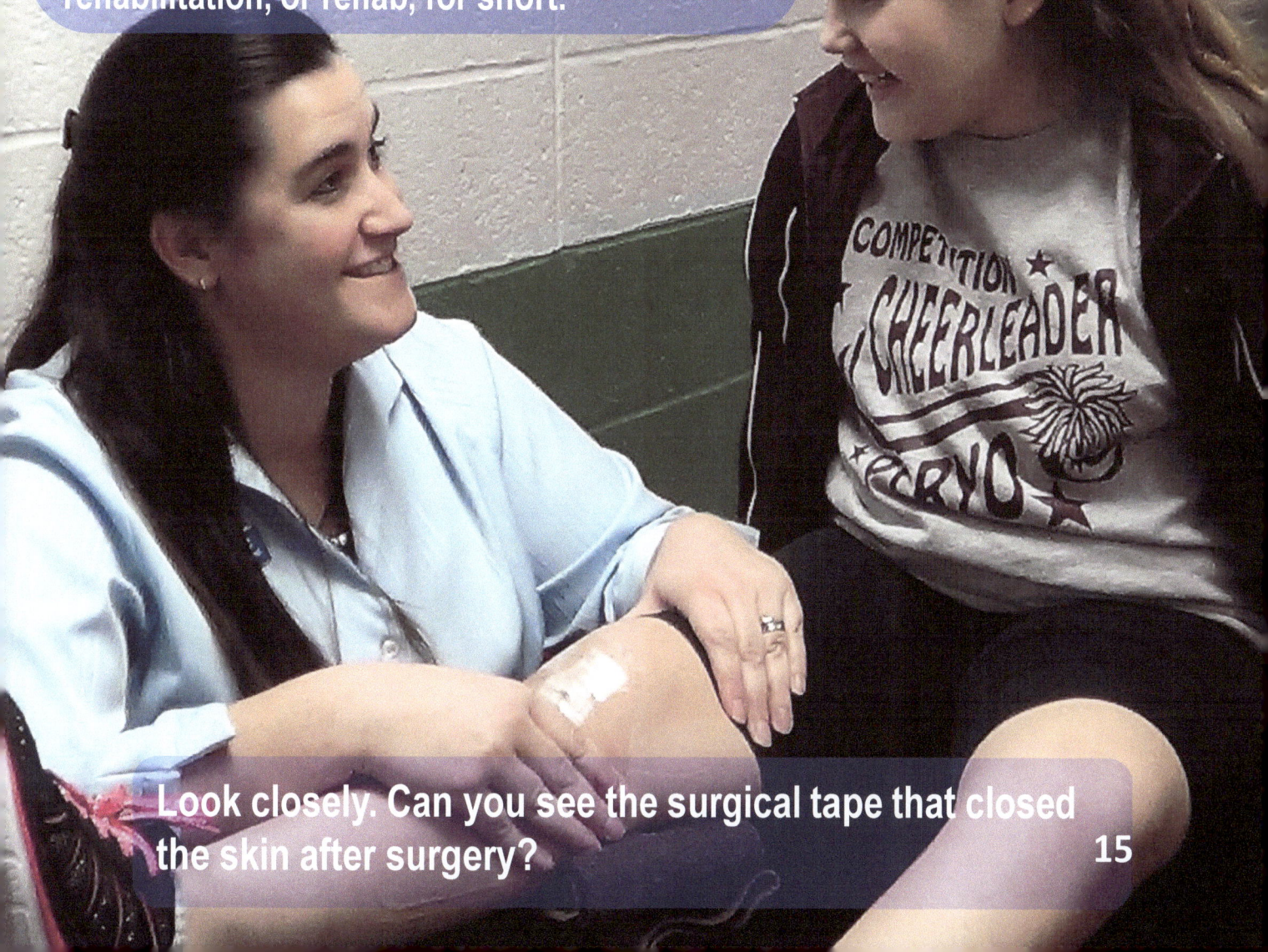

Look closely. Can you see the surgical tape that closed the skin after surgery?

Athletic trainers are very smart. These athletic trainers used their special knowledge to invent products that help children.

This athletic trainer invented a pad that protects people who have a special box called a pacemaker. The pacemaker helps their hearts to beat well.

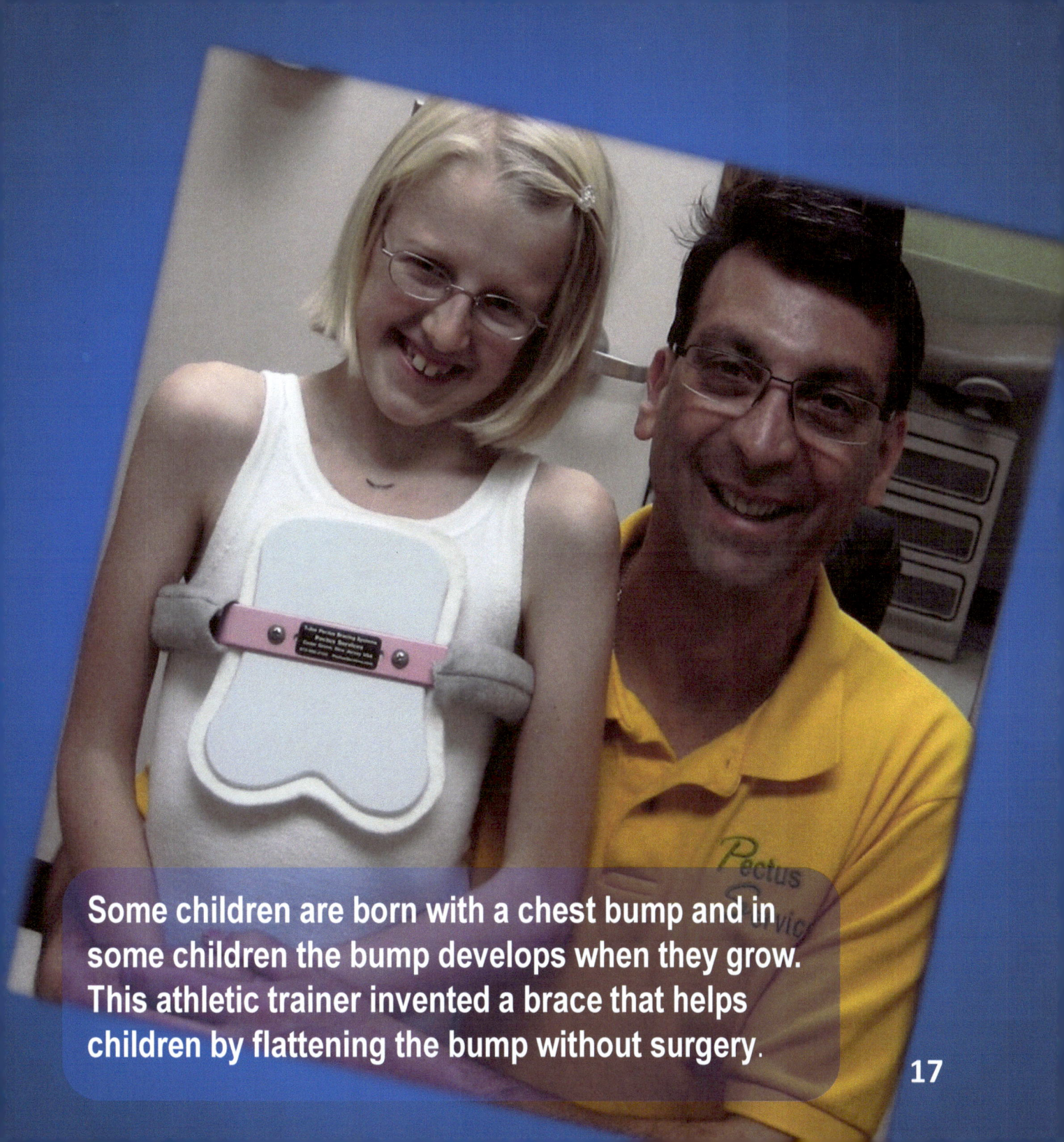

Some children are born with a chest bump and in some children the bump develops when they grow. This athletic trainer invented a brace that helps children by flattening the bump without surgery.

This tennis player is performing one of the tests that athletic trainers use after an athlete has had a concussion. Brain health is important for athletes of all ages.

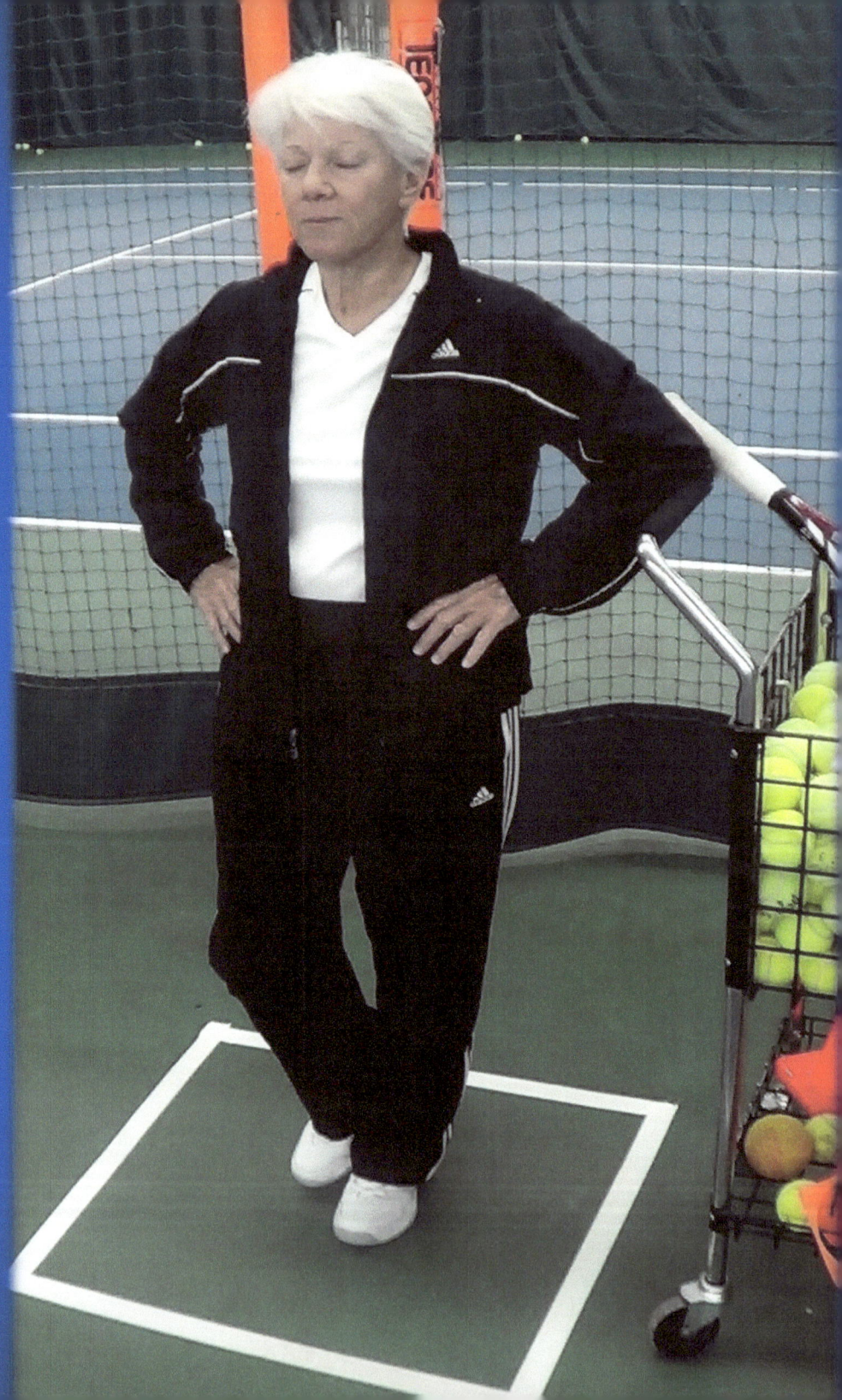

Rodeo athletes travel every week to compete. Managing their injuries is very challenging.

Special tape is used by athletic trainers to support joints so athletes can stay active while they heal. This tape is stretchy and strong.

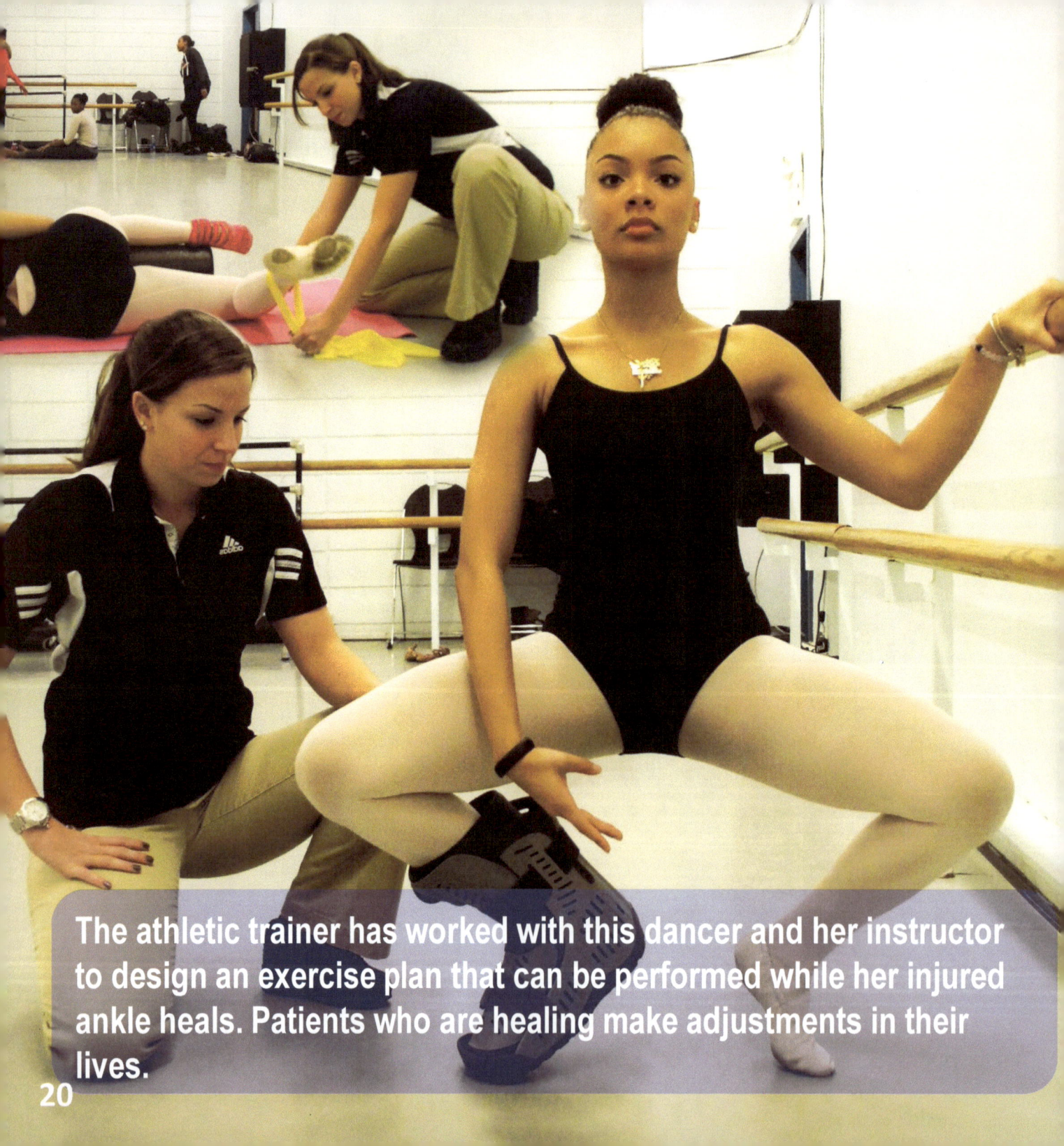

The athletic trainer has worked with this dancer and her instructor to design an exercise plan that can be performed while her injured ankle heals. Patients who are healing make adjustments in their lives.

People who do not move, see or hear like other people can be athletic trainers or patients of athletic trainers. They can do almost anything, they just might do it differently.

This paralympic athlete is explaining how he makes his racing gloves to his athletic trainer.

21

The athletic trainer is teaching this patient an exercise to strengthen the muscles that control her kneecap. People with different abilities make adjustments in the way they do things to reach their goals.

Athletic trainers keep notes and records on the health and treatments of all their patients. Sometimes they use paper and pencil, sometimes the computer and sometimes both.

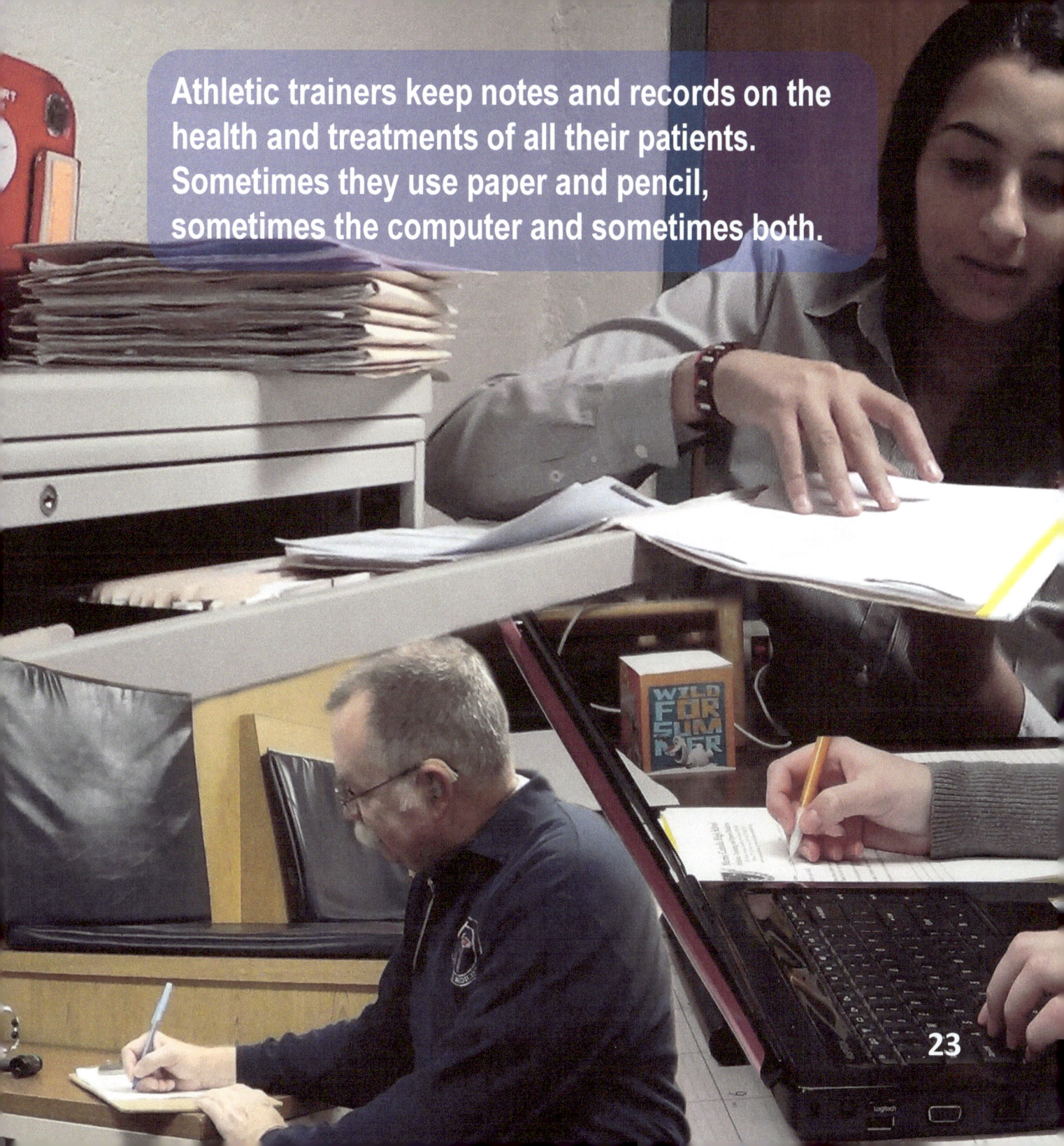

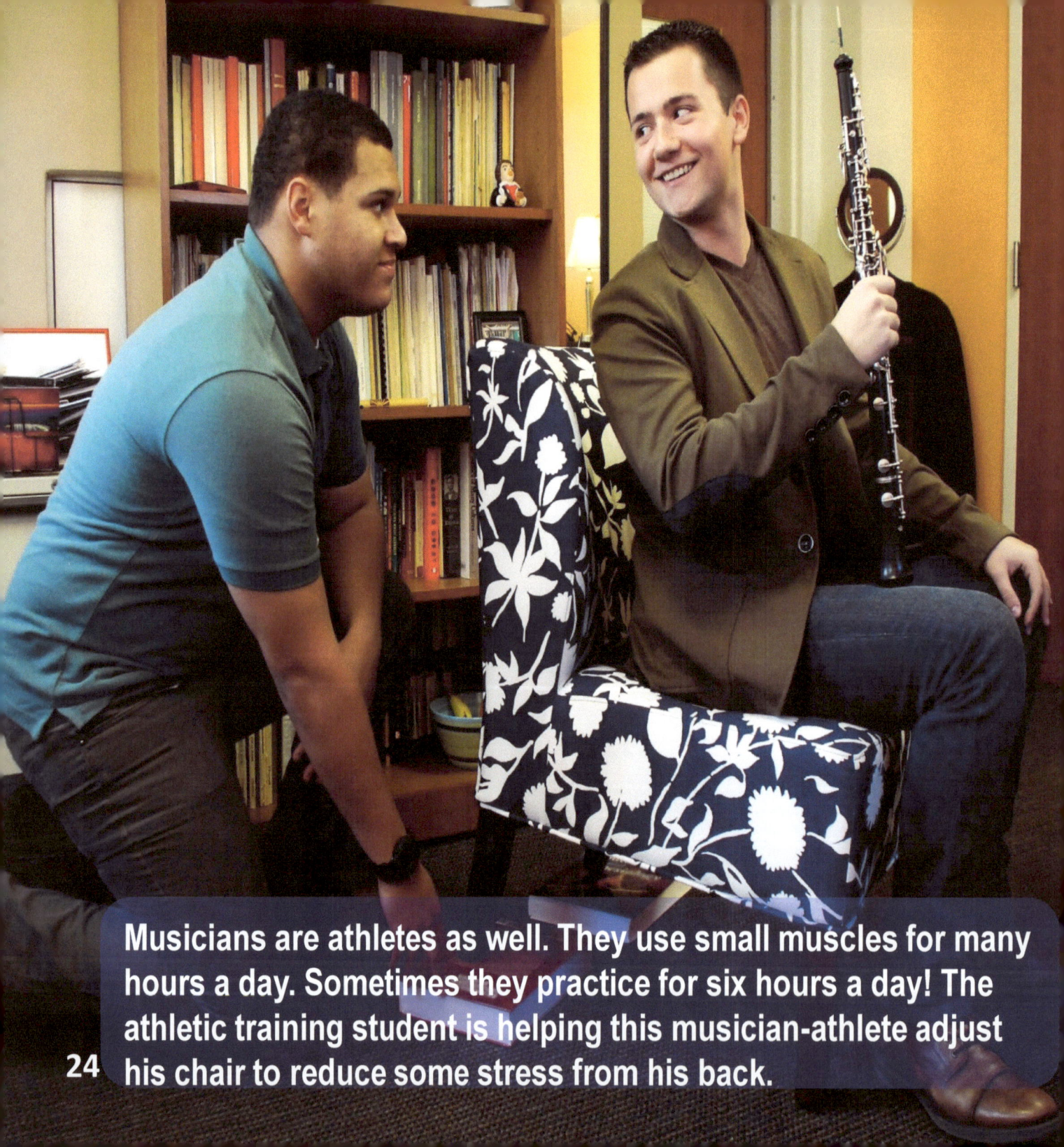

Musicians are athletes as well. They use small muscles for many hours a day. Sometimes they practice for six hours a day! The athletic training student is helping this musician-athlete adjust his chair to reduce some stress from his back.

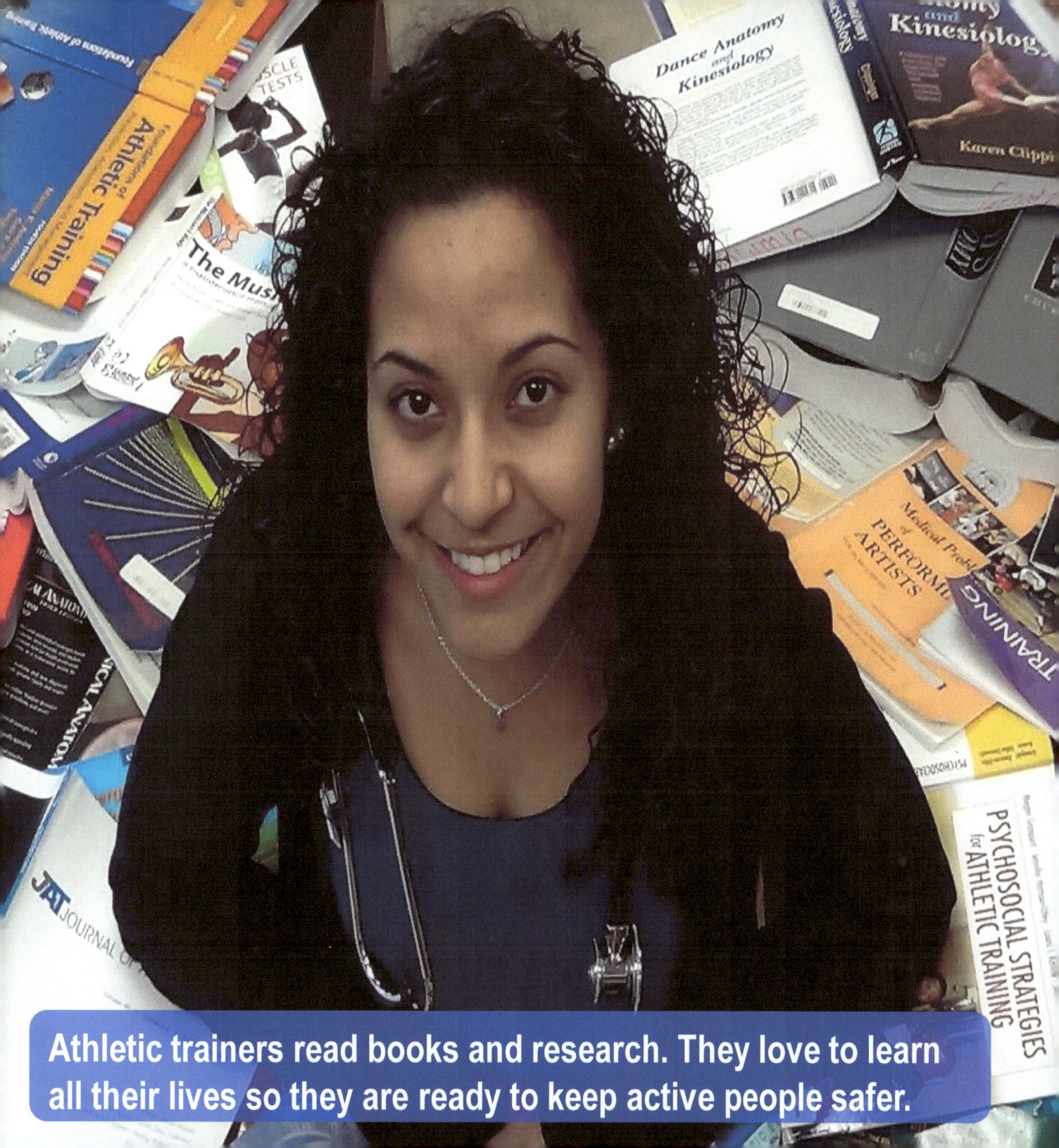

Athletic trainers read books and research. They love to learn all their lives so they are ready to keep active people safer.

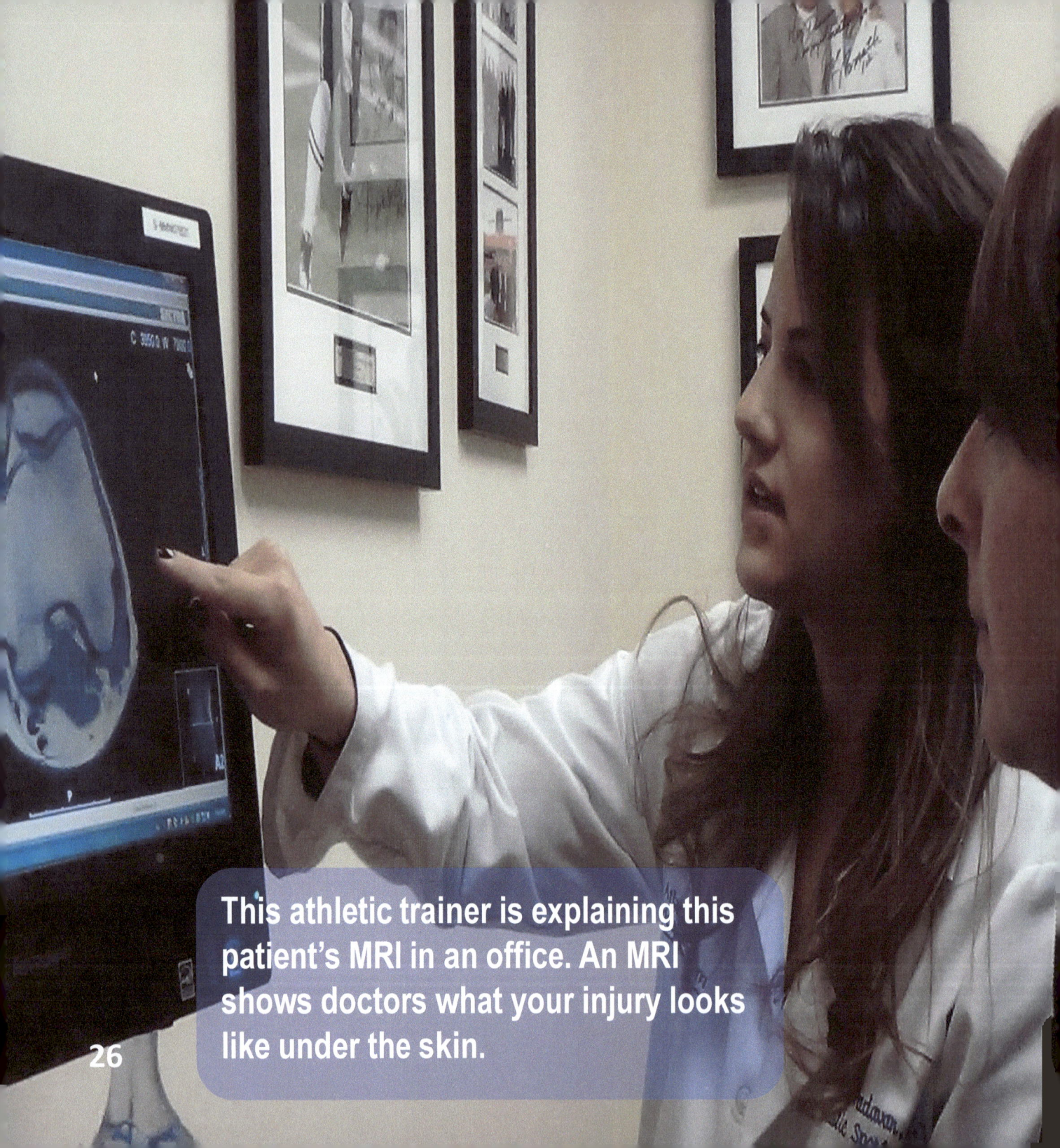

This athletic trainer is explaining this patient's MRI in an office. An MRI shows doctors what your injury looks like under the skin.

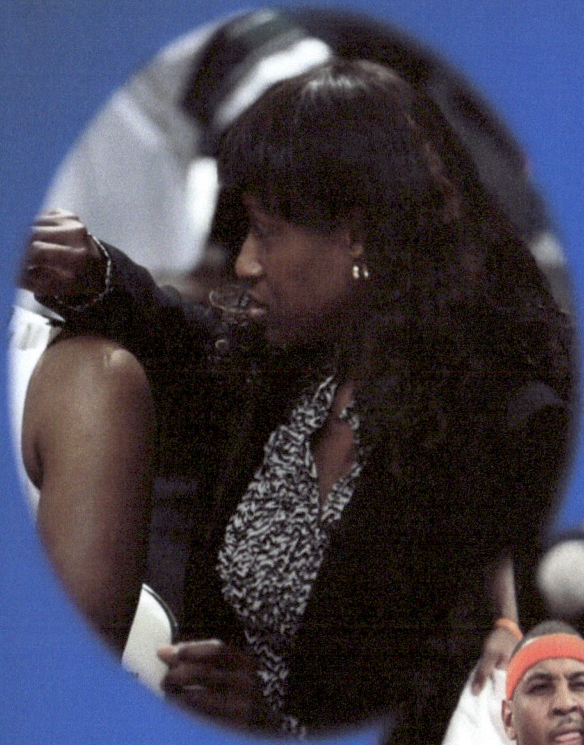

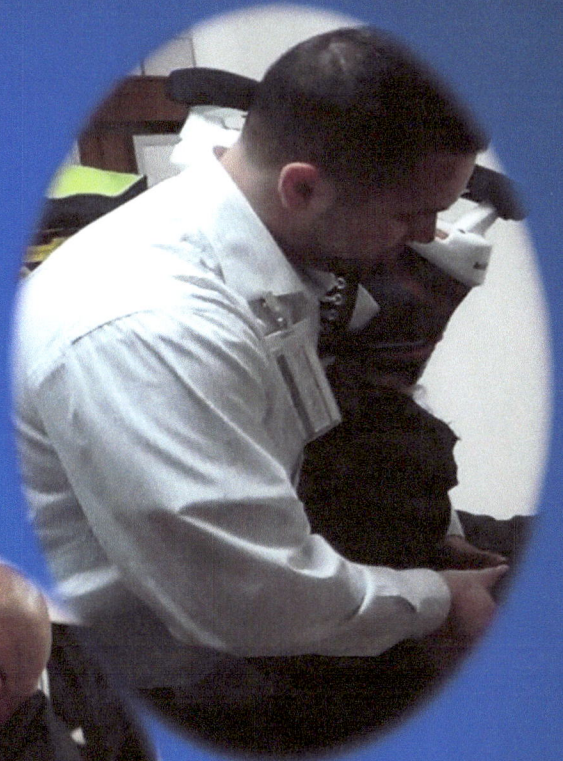

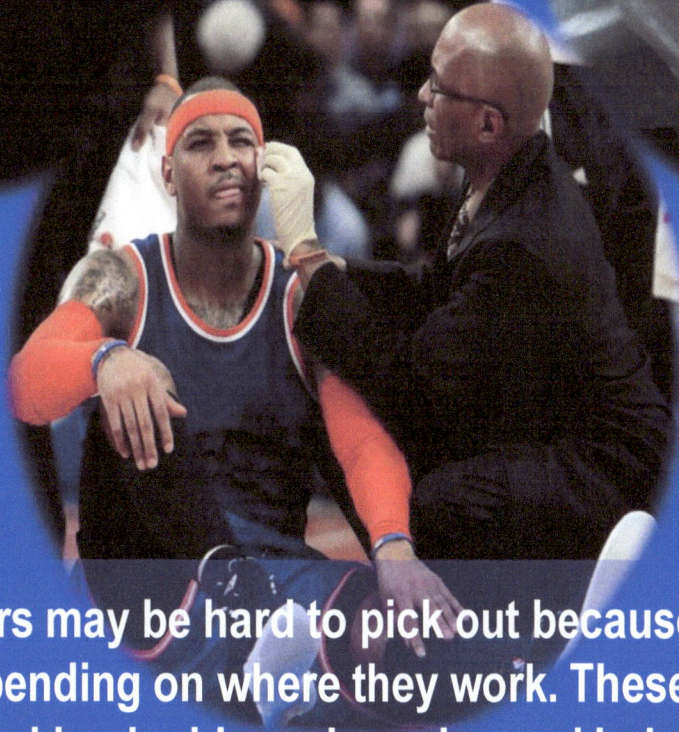

Athletic trainers may be hard to pick out because they dress differently depending on where they work. These athletic trainers are working inside and are dressed in business clothing.

27

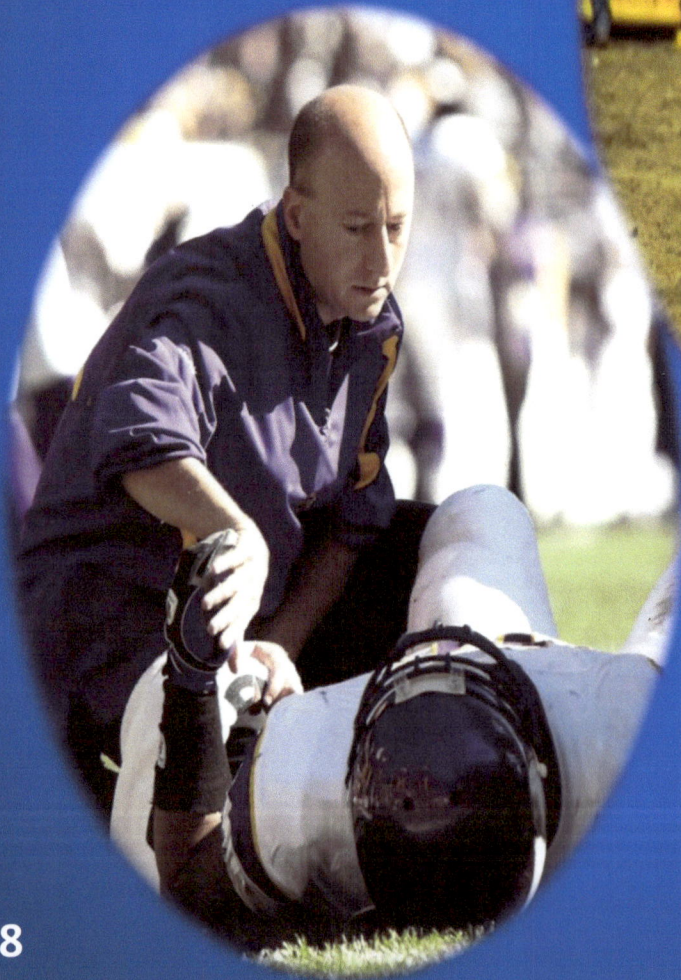

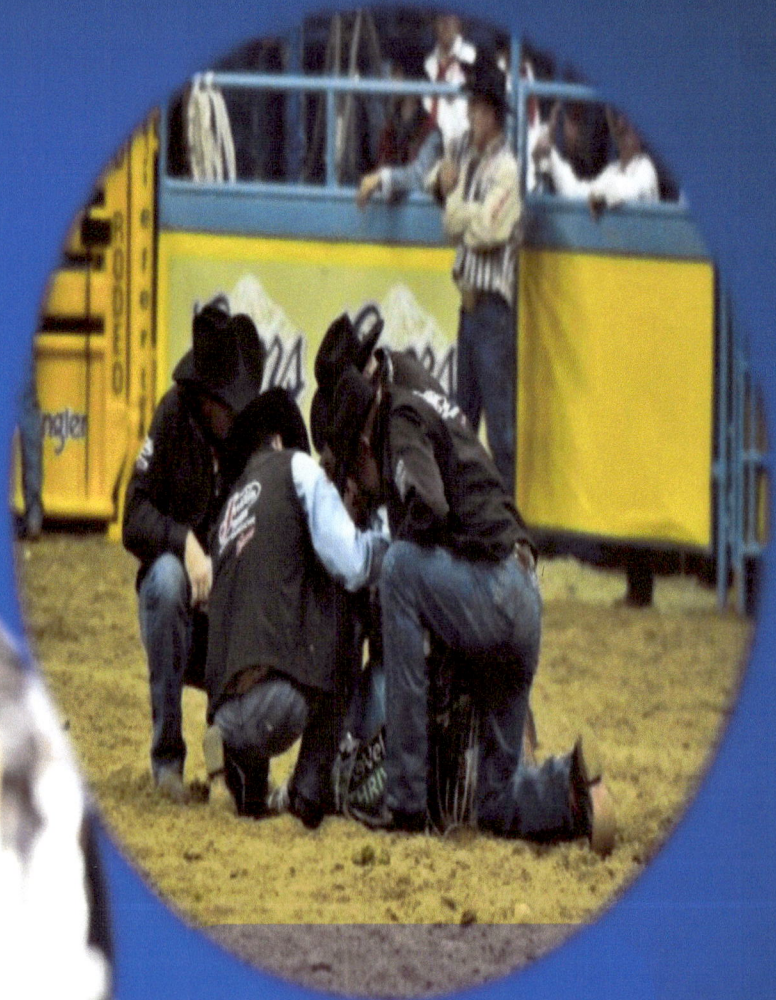

When they work outside, their clothing sometimes blends in with what the athletes wear.

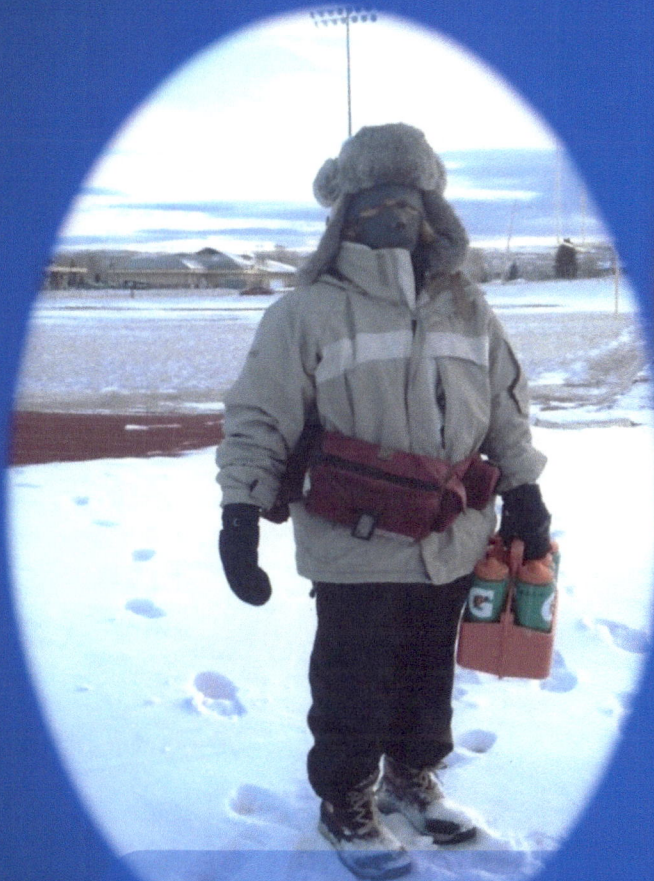

This athletic trainer works in Wyoming where part of the fall season is very cold.

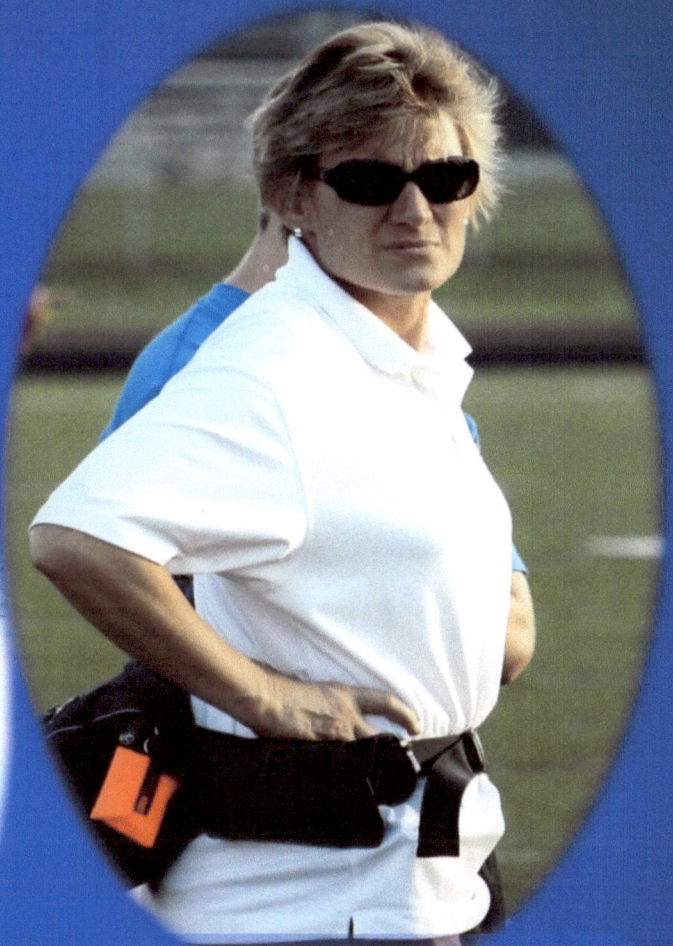

This athletic trainer works in Kansas where part of the fall season is very hot.

29

This athletic trainer wears scrubs when his job gets a little messy in the laboratory.

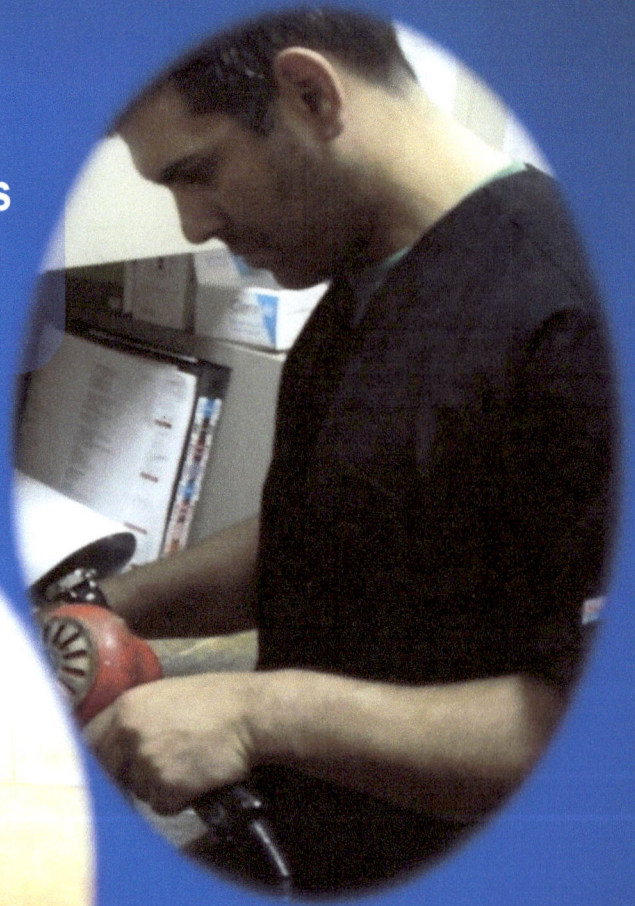

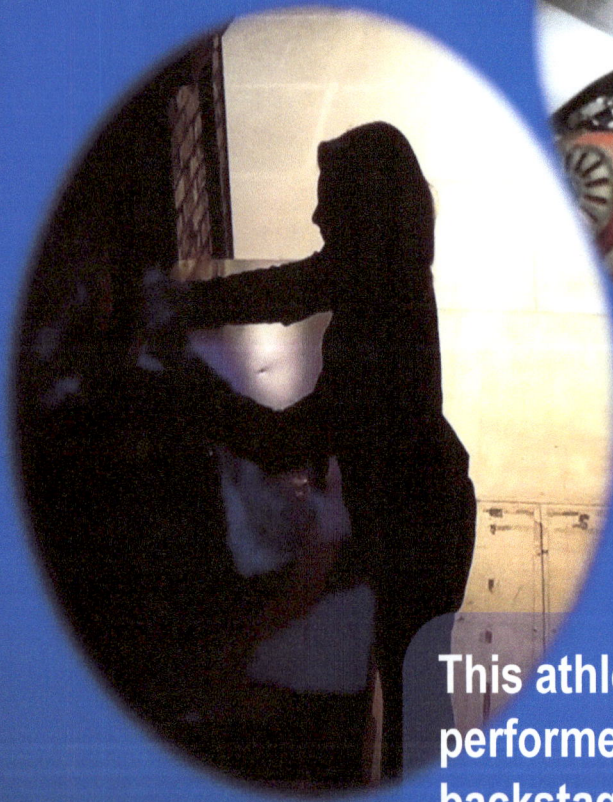

This athletic trainer works with performers. She is wearing black backstage so she will not stand out if she is accidentally seen by the audience.

Medical kit

Ice bag

gloves

Sling bag

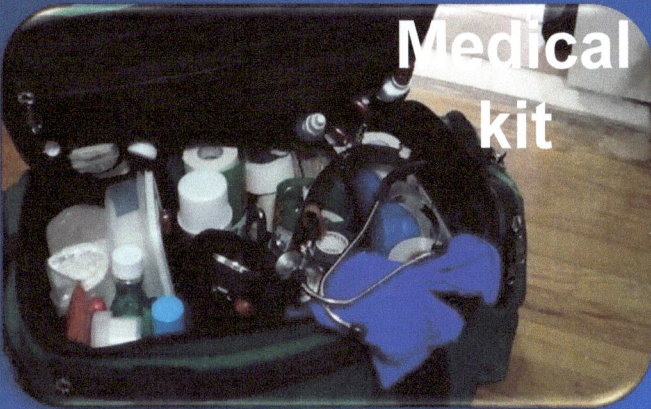

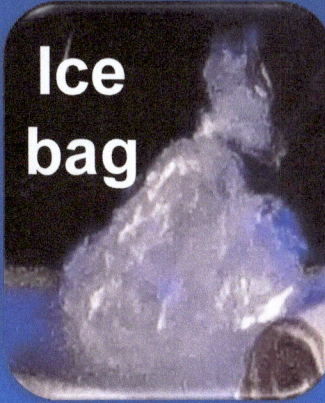

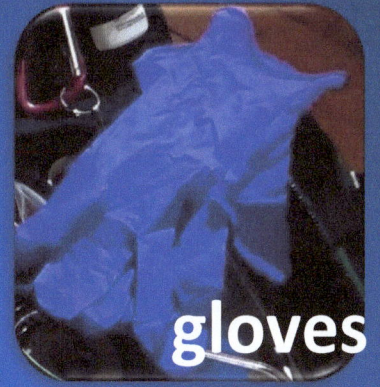

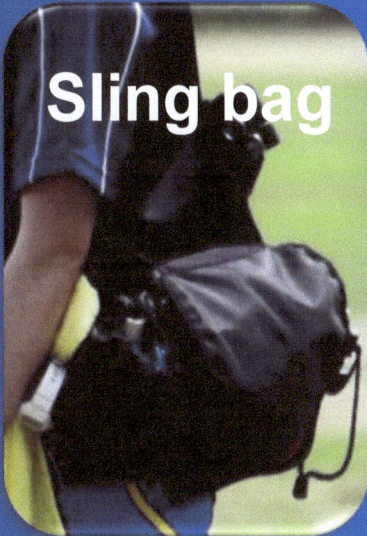

Athletic trainers use these things when they work. Can you find athletic trainers using these in this book?

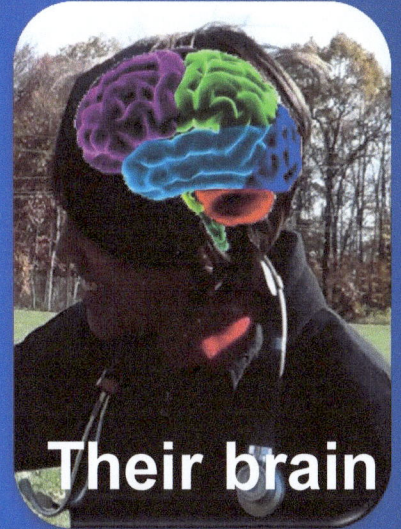

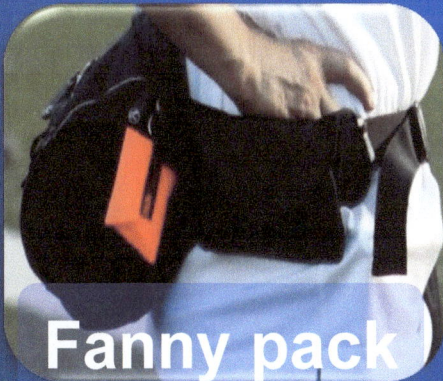

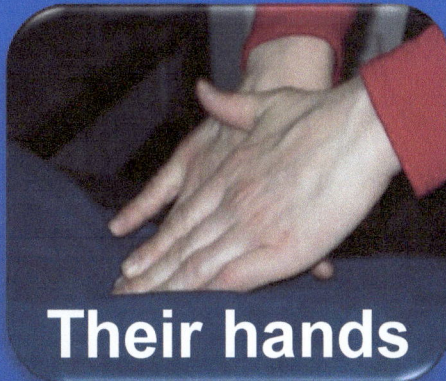

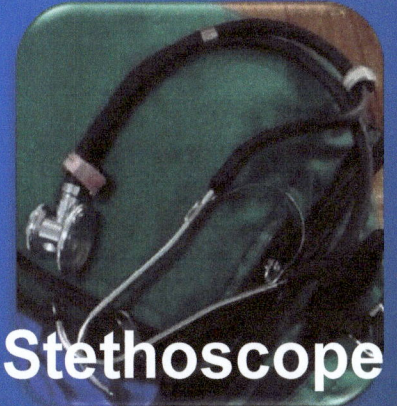

Their brain

Fanny pack

Their hands

Stethoscope

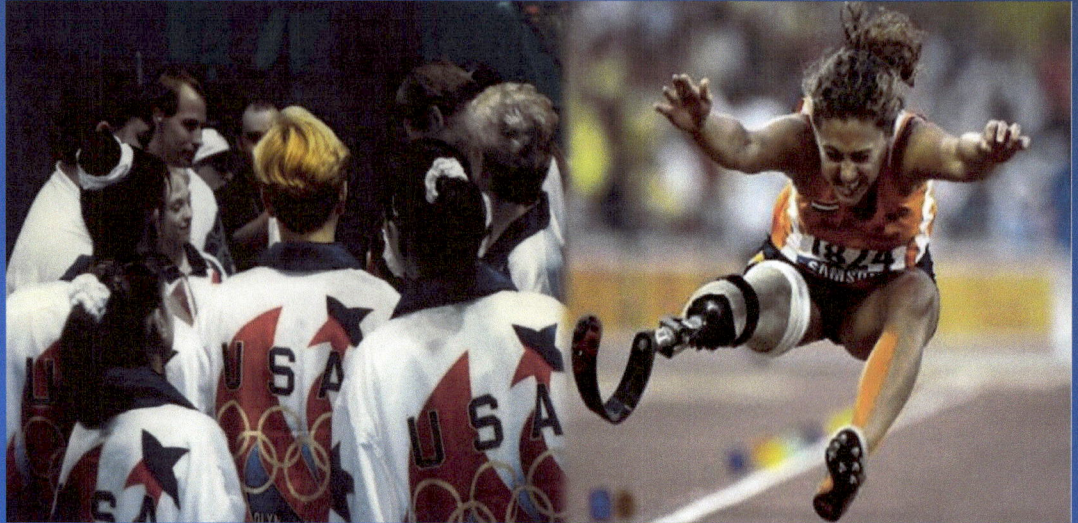

Athletic trainers also change people's lives in their free time. They volunteer professionally for athletic events like the Olympic and Paralympics,

Aiden

JDRF Walk

Aiden's Musketeers

Special Olympics

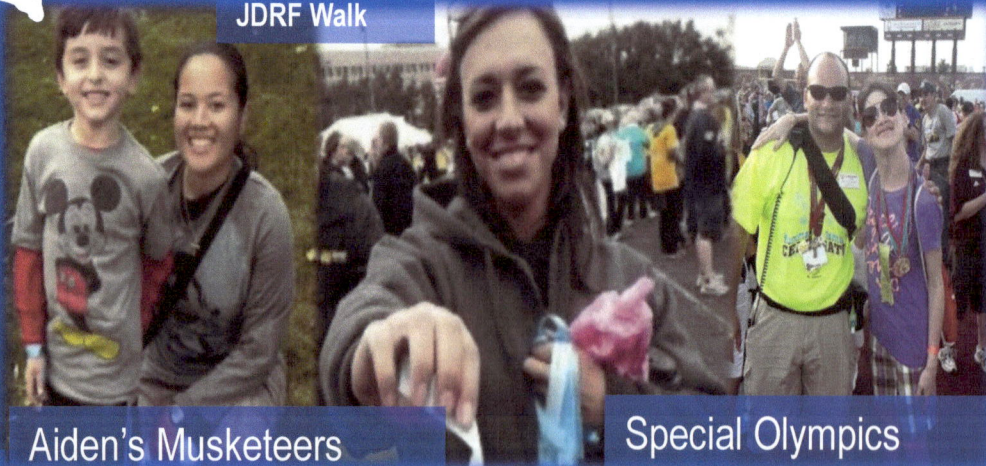

but their hearts are especially BIG for causes that help kids like the Juvenile Diabetes Research Foundation and Special Olympics.

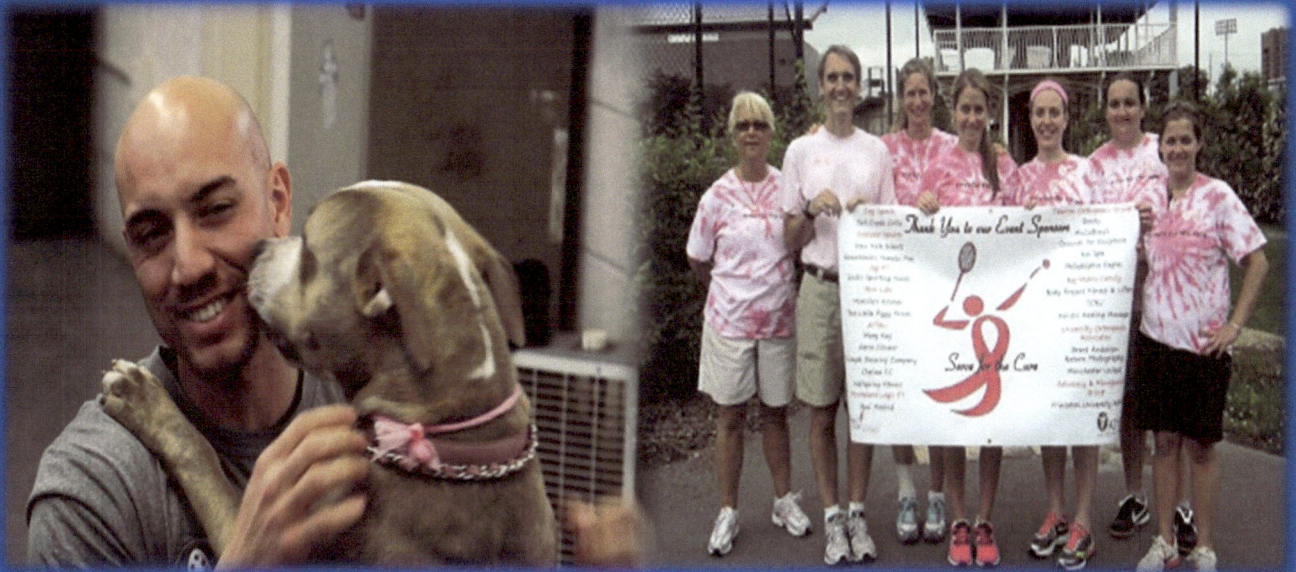

They make their communities better by volunteering for many causes like breast cancer and animal groups.

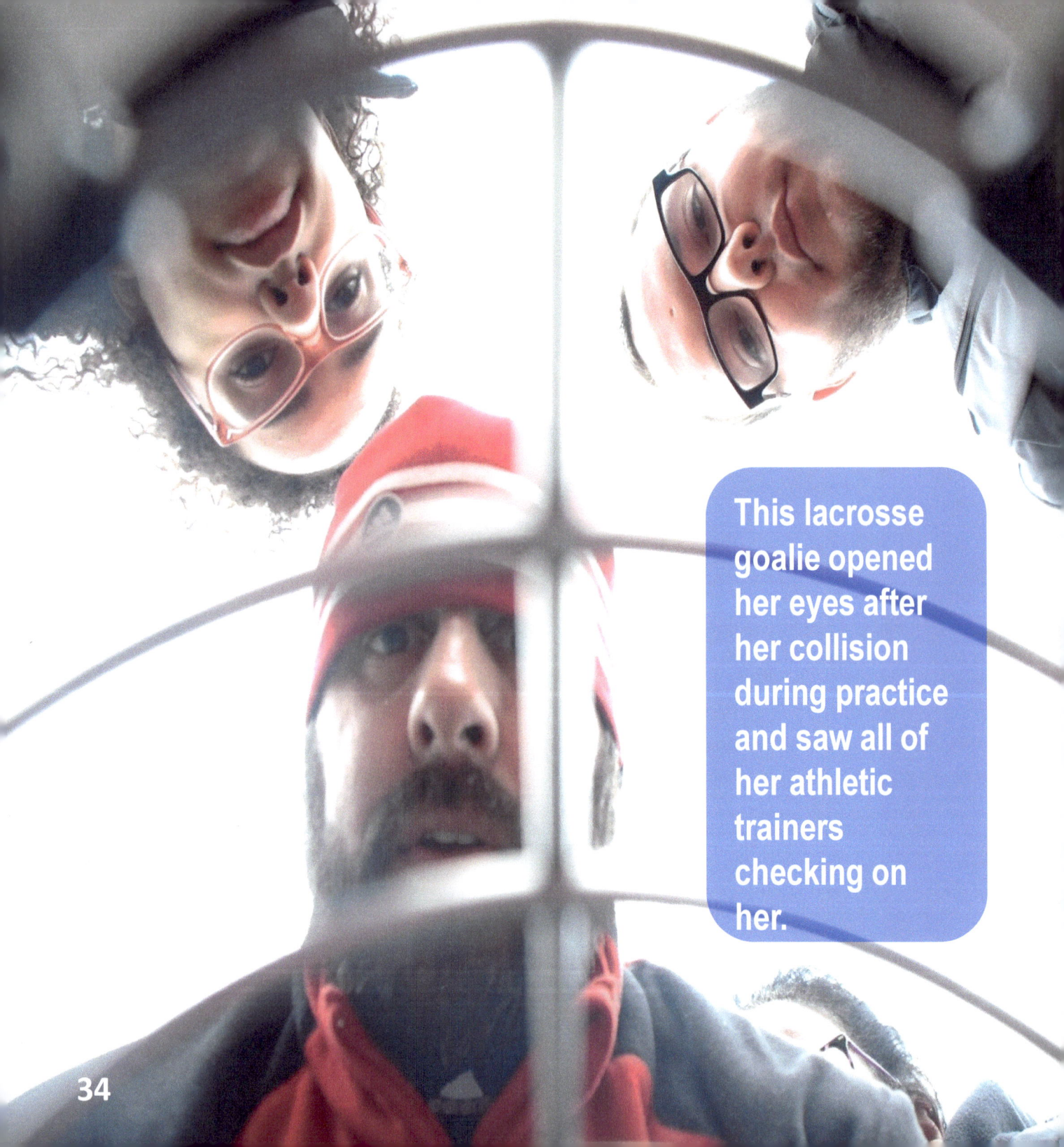

This lacrosse goalie opened her eyes after her collision during practice and saw all of her athletic trainers checking on her.

The athletic trainers place her onto a spine board to keep her spine safe until she arrives at the emergency room.

Athletic trainers also think ahead and try to prevent things from going wrong. If things go wrong anyway, they are calm in a crisis and solve problems well.

Athletic trainers help people get better with different treatments. Sometimes the treatments are things athletic trainers do to the patient, like using their hands to treat muscle pain.

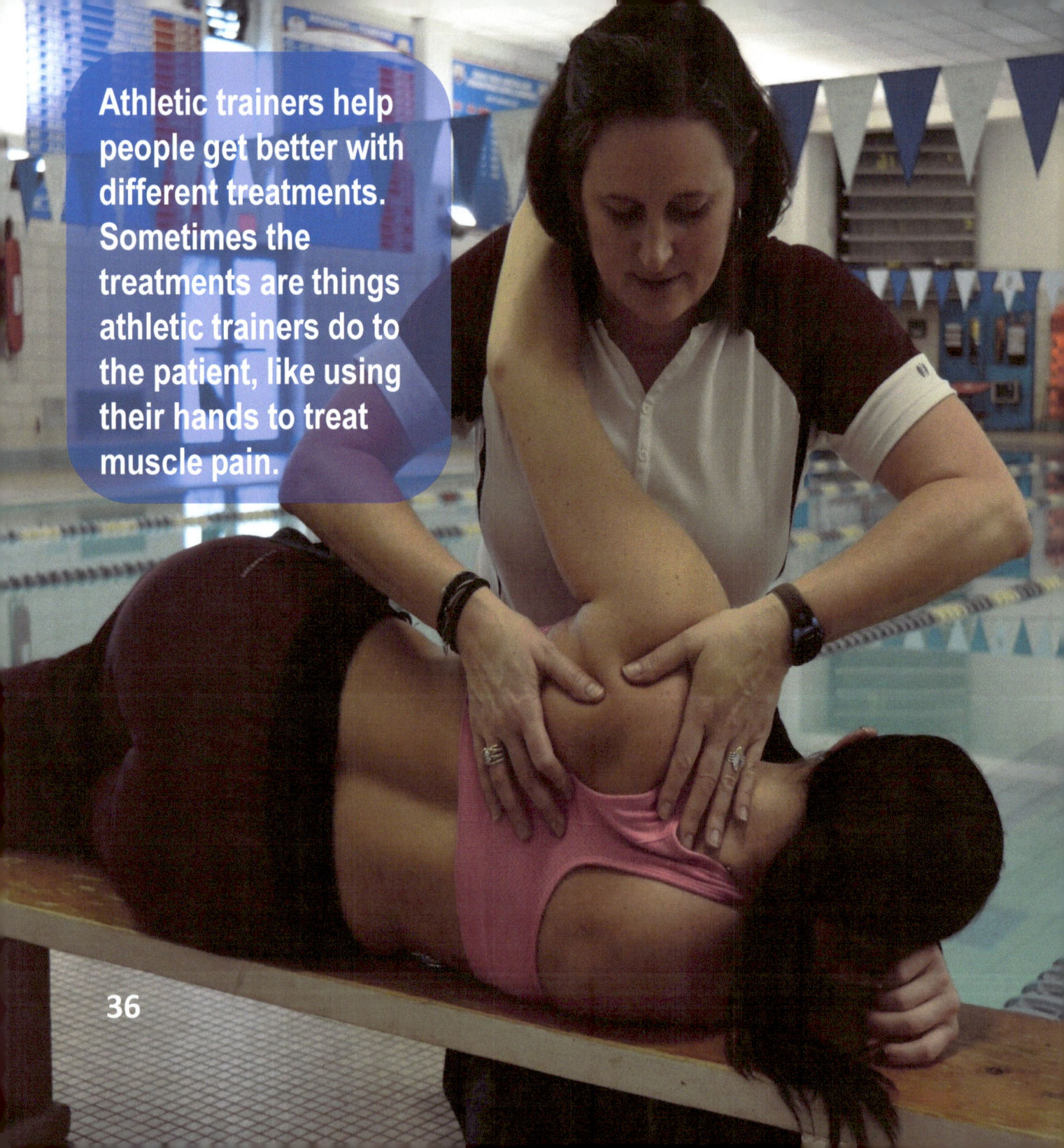

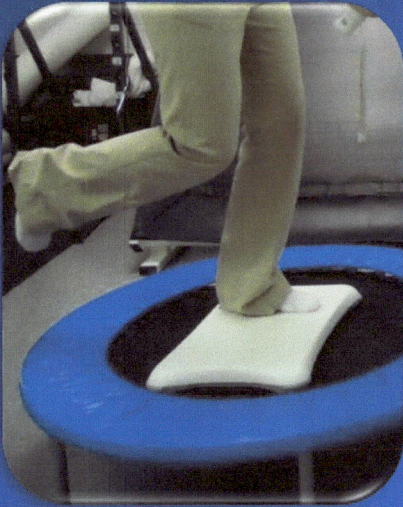

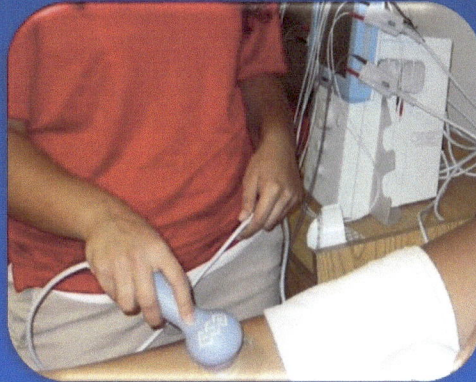

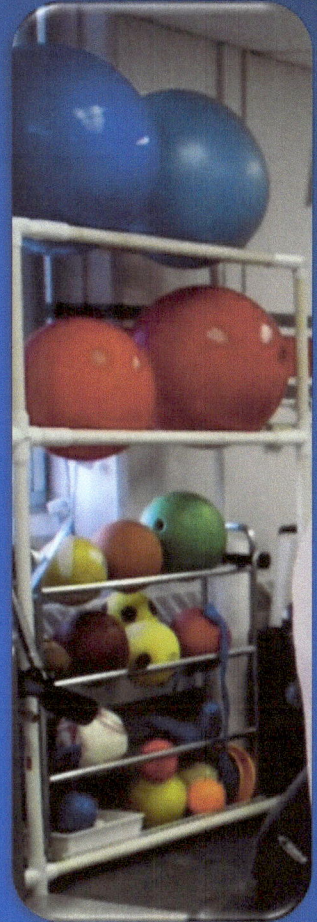

Sometimes athletic trainers use machines or other equipment.

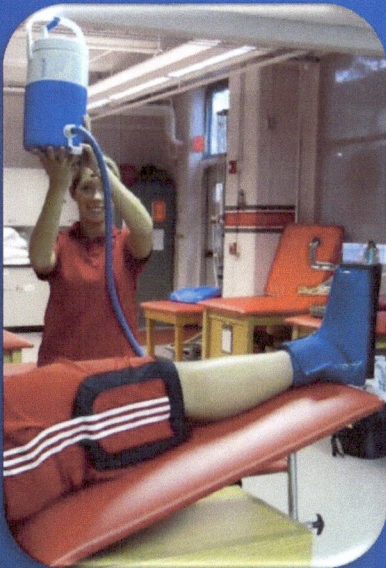

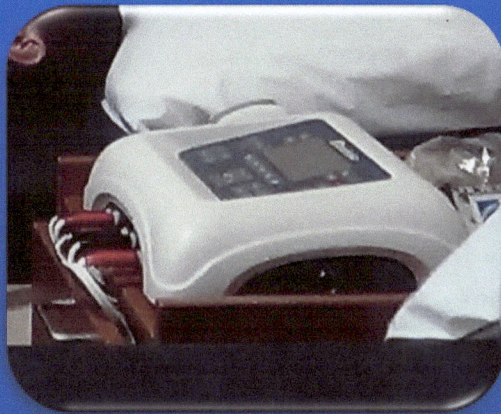

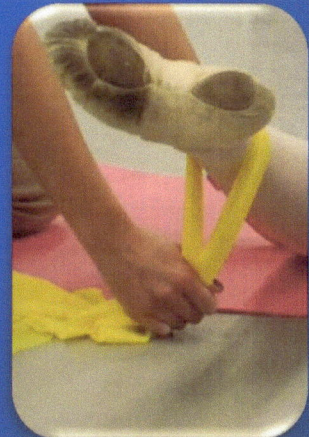

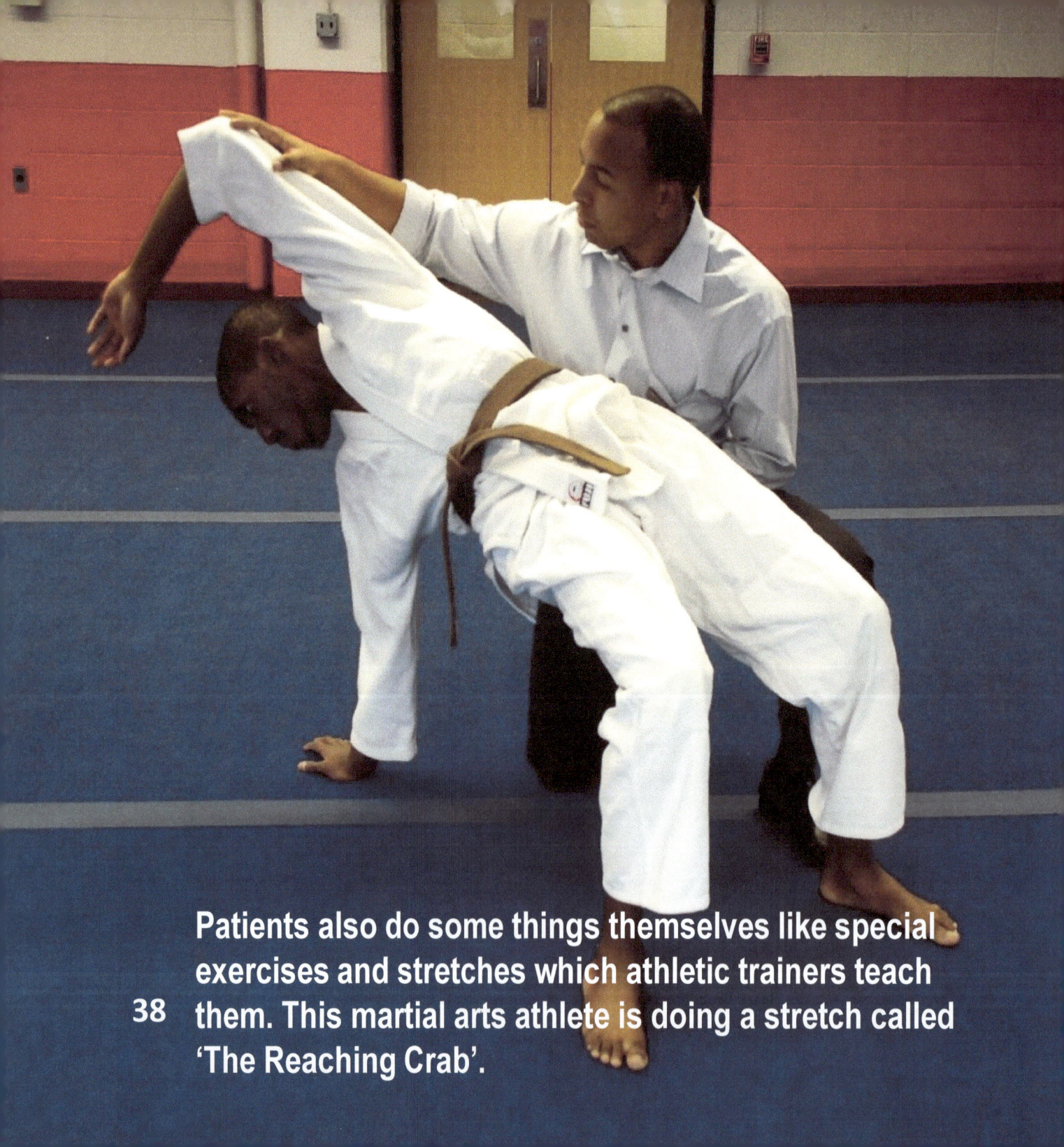

Patients also do some things themselves like special exercises and stretches which athletic trainers teach them. This martial arts athlete is doing a stretch called 'The Reaching Crab'.

38

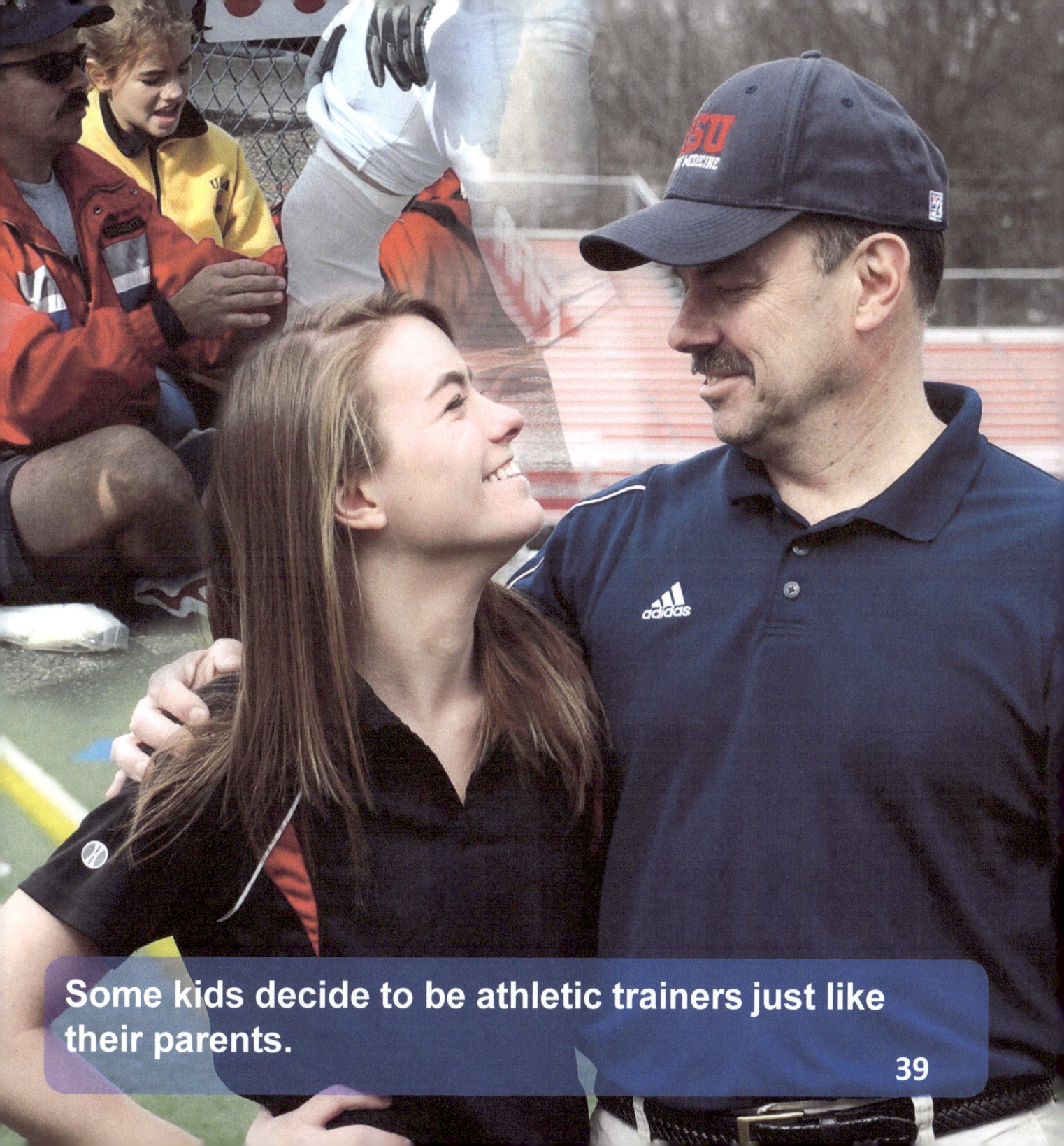

Some kids decide to be athletic trainers just like their parents.

To learn more about
the profession of
athletic training visit
www.nata.org

www.ingramcontent.com/pod-product-compliance
Lightning Source LLC
Chambersburg PA
CBHW052055190326
41519CB00002BA/238